The Health Secrets
of a
Naturopathic Doctor

The Health Secrets

of a

Naturopathic Doctor

M. O. Garten, D.C.

Parker Publishing Company, Inc.   West Nyack, N. Y.

© 1967, BY

PARKER PUBLISHING COMPANY, INC.

WEST NYACK, N. Y.

ALL RIGHTS RESERVED. NO PART OF THIS
BOOK MAY BE REPRODUCED IN ANY FORM OR
BY ANY MEANS, WITHOUT PERMISSION IN
WRITING FROM THE PUBLISHER.

LIBRARY OF CONGRESS
CATALOG CARD NUMBER: 67-15170

PRINTED IN THE UNITED STATES OF AMERICA
B & P

Dedication

It is said that a woman can either make or break a man. This could be carried further by declaring that some of us men would have gone down the drain a long time ago if it hadn't been for the strength and help of some unusual members of the *weaker sex*.

One runs out of adjectives attempting to describe the various faculties attached to these rare specimens of our female companions. Being wise, imbued with intuition, untiring in their endless work, yet sometimes delightfully capricious or pert, they keep going in the face of tremendous odds yet always maintaining grace, dignity and charm along with patience and dedication.

There are three words that express the true meaning of our thoughts regarding this exciting womanhood that makes life enchanting. With each new day granting another precious experience of togetherness I humbly say, *GOD BLESS THEM.*

I dedicate this book to one of the finest specimens in this category, my wife, Eva Garten, who inspired the writings but without her help the book could not have come into existence.

M. O. GARTEN, D.C.

Also by the Author

The Cycle of Health

Tomorrow's Health

The Dynamics of Vibrant Health and Neuropractic

Introduction

The words "aches and pains" are household terms in American life. In newspapers, magazines, on radio and the screen, we are constantly reminded of it. And no wonder! More than nine out of ten Americans are sick. This figure, of course, includes those of us, who as yet do not show the disease in a demonstrable form. Yet, nearly half, or 44.9 percent of the flower of our manhood is unfit for military service.

A great part of man's attention has been taken up with this business of aches and pains. There are many ways and means in which they can be overcome as there are "many roads leading to Rome."

The way to health as covered in this book does not point to short cuts. But it does indicate the shortest route to better health.

Aches and pains are messages indicating the presence of disorders in the living organism. The removal of such signals, without overcoming its causes, brings no lasting solution to the problem.

Where there is smoke, there is fire. Let us not only get at the smoke, *but* also actually *put out the fire*.

I have spent a lifetime treating disease, as well as teaching the profession of drugless healing. My activities were carried out in the Americas, Europe and Asia.

Practically every existing healing system had been tried and tested by me. If the method worked, it would be used; if not, discarded. Speed, efficiency and scientific fundamentals were the bases of my judgment.

The suggestions offered in this book can produce improvements in the recovery from any diseases. Aches and pains will disappear and once more life becomes permeated with joy and excitement, brimming with vitality!

M. O. GARTEN, D.C.

Notice: Do not purchase this book with the hopes of curing cancer or any other chronic disease.

We offer it for informative purposes to help cope with health situations and do not claim this book furnishes information as to an effective treatment or cure of the disease discussed—according to currently accepted *medical* opinion.

Although it is your right to adopt your own dietary and treating pattern, nevertheless suggestions offered in this book should not be applied to a specific individual except by his doctor who would be familiar with individual requirements and any possible complications. Never attempt a lengthy fast without competent professional supervision.

Contents

3. ACHES AND PAINS RELIEVED WITH THE FAST
(Continued)

4. FOOD—ITS RELATIONS TO ACHES AND PAINS 91

1

How to Get Relief from Pains and Aches without Drugs

The word pain comes from the Latin *poena*—meaning penality—punishment.

In Greek we find *poine*—meaning penality.

A dictionary defines *pain* as denoting sharp, sometimes sudden suffering, *ache*, a continuous, often dull bodily pain; it can also be described as:

1. A form of consciousness characterized by desire of escape or avoidance, and varying from slight uneasiness to extreme distress or torture.

2. An affection or feeling proceeding from a derangement of function, disease or bodily injury.

Pain is usually caused by an agent that damages or threatens to destroy body structures or the organism as a whole.

So much for the negative aspects of pain. What about its positive side? The old adage about *pain being an angel in disguise* assumes more concrete proportions the more we acquaint ourselves with its many manifestations.

Primarily, it must be emphasized that pain is not only a distinct separable sensation but is undoubtedly the most primitive device for self-preservation and protection from bodily harm.

Pain can be classified according to the region of its location or by the quality of the experience. We find cutaneous (skin) pain, deep pain from muscles, tendons and joints, visceral pain from internal organs, and referred pain. *Superficial Pain* is transmitted through tiny nerve endings called spots, as are other skin sensory nerves. The pain spots far outnumber all other "spots" put together, as would be expected from their protective function.

The whole human skin has some 30,000 warm spots, 200,000 cold spots, 500,000 touch spots but as many as 3,000,000 **pain** spots. Pain spots are more numerous at the roots of limbs. **Per** square centimeter on the palm, soles and the tip of the **nose,** there are 40-70 pain spots, while in the armpit there are about 200.

Deep Pain is caused by some degenerating or harmful change in muscle, tendon or joints. The exact location by Orthodox method is difficult to ascertain but is becoming increasingly positive by the use of "Neuropractic."

Visceral Pain is localized in particular organs. Hunger pains are usually felt in the region of the stomach. Heart pains are frequently localized directly under the breastbone.

Referred Pain is usually caused by some damage sustained by an internal organ, but referred by the nervous system to a superficial, sometimes distant location.

Angina pectoris, a pain in the chest caused by spasmatic contraction (cholesterol infusion) of the coronary arteries of the heart, is frequently referred to the left shoulder and arms as well as under left side of left breast. Liver abnormalities may be referred to the back of right shoulder.

NEUROPRACTIC—A NEW APPROACH
TO BODY DISORDERS

The practice of Neuropractic may be applied in most cases of body disorders.

In a hypothetical case of backache, the offending nerve tissues are located and found to be congested, "ropy," rigid and reacting extremely painful to the touch.

Pressure applications are given, with the patient feeling gratified about the "discovery" of cause of a certain abnormal or painful region. This gratified feeling is evident even though the patient feels a cutting or other pain sensation during pressure manipulations.

Within a relative, short period, from 2 to 15 minutes, mysteriously most pain disappears and affected nerve areas regain an elastic and smooth characteristic.

This is not all. The respective anatomical segments which were connected to the treated nerves, also respond with favorable improvement. In case of kidney disorders, the patient will soon notice more efficient functions. When motor nerves are involved (legs, arms, etc.), the patient is now enabled to make better use of these body parts.

THE "BALL" TREATMENT

Quite often it is impossible to procure the help of an operator skilled in Neuropractic.

Balls of several sizes can come to the rescue—particularly also, if one wishes to treat himself.

The balls are made out of rubber or plastics, are semi-rigid and can be purchased in most stores where children's toys are sold.

Three sizes have been found to be effective 3-, 2- and 1-inch in diameter. (Figure 1)

It is best to lie on floor covered with carpet, rug or blanket. The surface must be relatively hard, that is why the floor best answers the purpose. (Bed or couch is too soft.)

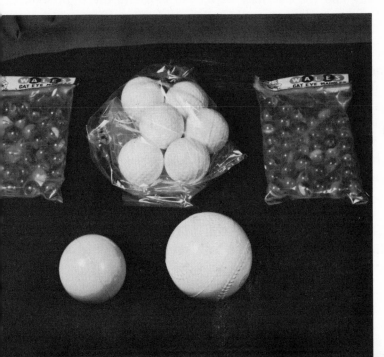

Figure 1

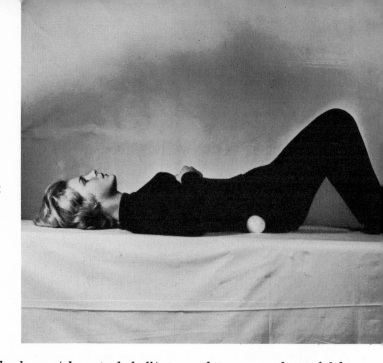

Figure 2

The large (three-inch ball) is used in cases of painful hip conditions. Lie on the back or affected side and insert ball directly *under* painful area.

In some severe cases it may be too painful to move the ball into the exact spot. In such a circumstance, place the ball as near as can be endured to the area of pain. In a matter of a few minutes, it will be found that the pain sensations are lessening and the ball may be moved closer to the right spot. (Figure 2)

In this way, one or several "approaching" movements may have to be made to arrive at the exact location.

The smaller balls (2- or 1-inch in diameter) have proven to be efficient in pain area of upper back. In this category we find typical heart or liver afflictions, kidney abnormalities and frequently nerve strangulations to adrenal glands.

It was found that the smaller (1-inch size) ball was more practical in the upper back, while the larger ones (2-and 3-inch in diameter) answered the purpose in lower back and hip.

Also, it was discovered that in upper back several small balls (between 5 and 8) held together in a sack of cloth, "worked" muscle and nerves more efficiently. (Figure 3)

The location of the ball or balls should be slightly changed in intervals of two minutes or so.

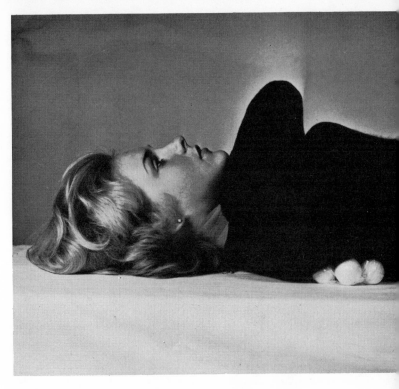

Figure 3

The entire treatment in one single area need not take more time than 15 minutes. If more than one body area is involved, the entire treatment may take one hour, not oftener than every other day.

THE MARBLE TREATMENT

A number of European health resorts made it mandatory to their patients to walk part of the time barefooted on coarse sand, wet grass or fine gravel. The purpose of this walking exercise is to stimulate or "pressurize" the soles of feet containing numerous nerve endings.

As indicated in these pages, certain interactions of the general nervous system bring about definite reflex effects to organs situated in a distant area of the body.

Thus, eyes, ears, heart, kidneys, etc., can be favorably influenced through this stimulation or pressure subjection of the feet. Since it may be difficult to go without footwear in our large communities, the marble "treatment" has proven to be of merit.

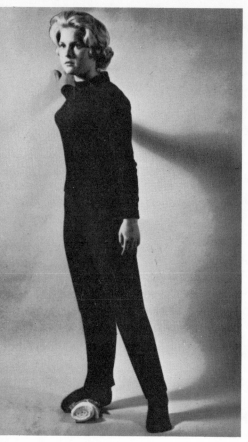

Figure 4

Figure 5

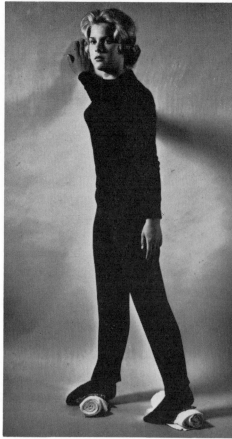

6

It is best to use bags of medium sized marbles (about ¾″ in diameter, generally sold forty in a plastic bag. (Figure 1)

Such a light covering is not strong enough for repeated use. It is suggested to re-enforce bag with one made out of canvas, heavy muslin or other fabric.

For most effective use, take bath towel and wrap tightly into roll. Place marble bag on this roll and step one foot at a time on top of marbles. Try to find painful regions which will receive primary consideration. It is best to hold on to a door frame while submitting to this "stepping treatment." First take one foot, then the other. The purpose of the towel roll is to permit the "pressurizing" of foot areas curving upward from bottom—such as the transverse arch. (Figure 4)

Start gently, if pain at beginning is too intense, shift part of body weight to other foot until full weight can be endured on marbles. In some cases it may be possible to place both feet on two separate bags of marbles. (Figure 5)

See Chart "A" on page 17 for reflex centers of feet.

THE CARPET "ROLL TREATMENT"

In the course of my teaching practice, I met an unusual, energetic, and enthusiastic man, being somewhere around ninety years "young."

This gentleman, an Osteopathic physician, is so wholeheartedly "sold" on the benefits derived from the use of a tightly wound roll, that the good doctor makes use of the contraption even when reclining in an armchair, watching television.

A wide board is inserted from the seat to the back of the chair, which now serves as the "floor" in providing a hard surface to contact the roll. The entire length of back is now gently rocked and twisted as outlined above.

The doctor appears to be in excellent health, is still practicing as a physician and insists that he intends to continue so for another twenty-five years.

The lively gentleman told me that his feelings of well-being had not always been the case in his past. When he was in his seventies, he had developed a curvature and rigidity in his spine. All movements became painful, and he had been forced to seek professional help from another doctor.

For the purpose of convenience and saving time, our good doctor had experimented with several devices to bring about self-treatment of the afflicted spine. After many trials, the carpet roll had been found to answer the purpose most efficiently. The physical basis of this treatment is the principle of the fulcrum.

The famous Greek philosopher Demosthenes made the statement: "Give me a fulcrum and I will move the world."

The spinal column is considered the *life line* of the body and as such should be preserved with emphasis on elasticity and movability. The customary forward bending and increasing stiffness of the spine is *not* necessarily a normal and unavoidable side effect of advanced age.

While we have become accustomed to accept such stiffenings and bendings as inevitable signs of senility, actual clinical experiences in hundreds of cases have proven the fact that such spinal changes of "old age" can be greatly slowed down, if not nearly prevented.

In the event of already established curvature and rigidity, it has been demonstrated that a decided improvement of such abnormalities can be achieved.

In this connection, we must somewhat refresh our memory with the anatomical make-up of the spine. Briefly, there are 24 distinct bony segments (bodies or vertebraes) separated or "cushioned" by discs.

These discs are soft, elastic, highly vascular (spongy) and intended by nature to act as "shock absorbers" to the vulnerable bone segments or bodies of the spine.

Now we are coming to a still more essential mechanism providing for maintenance of integrity to this most important framework of the body. Here we find muscles and nerves, highly integrated to exert an exact and equal amout of tension or pull on either side of the spine.

Since muscle tension (tonicity) is controlled by nerve stimulation for body movement, it is obvious that such muscle tension could become uneven, permitting the existence of higher tension on one side of the spine, with corresponding laxity on other side.

While general emphasis is usually accorded to the spine, we must not forget other nerve involvements such as the autonomic chains also being situated in the back.

Therefore, a tremendous physical response to these important regulators can be aroused by any force which can be applied in precise amounts.

The severity and extent of "treatment" is always under the control of the "patient" since it is self-given. Individual tolerance is a most unmistakable and trustworthy guide, rendering valuable protection for over-use.

CAUTION: For those afflicted with *Osteoporosis,* a disease denoting porosity or fragility of bones, it is best to first secure a check-up from their physician as in some severe cases bones may be as brittle as pretzels. Fortunately, such extreme cases are rare. It is advisable to always start very mildly with the exercises.

SURFACE REQUIREMENTS FOR ROLL EXERCISE

A semi-rigid surface is essential—bed or couch are too soft and will not work. The floor, covered with carpet or rug, seems best to answer the purpose.

TECHNIQUE OF "ROLL" EXERCISE

Place roll under upper shoulders, slightly below nape of neck. Both hands are interlocked and placed behind neck, below the skull. Arms are folded backward with head, neck and portions of back *above* roll being *twisted left and right* as far as can be comfortably tolerated for a few times.

In the second phase of exercise, we remain with folded hands under neck but *bring both arms together.*

The movement now becomes a rocking motion of head, neck and *upper* portion of back, *up and down.*

This exercise is also followed a few times (not more than two at the start), always beginning gently without arousing any feelings of discomfort or pain.

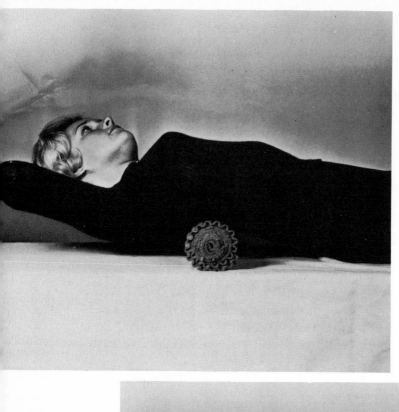

Figure 6

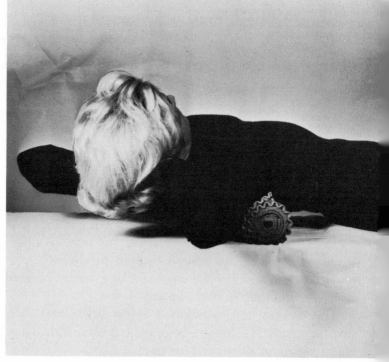

Figure 7

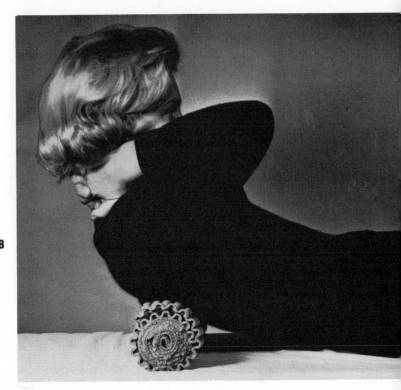

Figure 8

Having completed both movements, sideways and up and down, we proceed now to our next position by placing the roll about *one and one-half inch below former position.* In this manner, the next vertebrae will be encountered. *The side movement is made first, to be followed with the rocking up and down exercise.*

Having made these movements a few times, we proceed to the next position of vertebrae, footward.

PLACEMENT OF CARPET ROLL

The roll can be moved by lifting upper body and then sliding the freed roll to the next spot below. Also, in a more direct manner, the body is simply "scooted" on the roll a little to the next position, the roll acting literally as a "roll."

FULCRUM PRINCIPLE

Definition of fulcrum: The point about which a lever turns while transmitting a force. The crowbar is a typical example

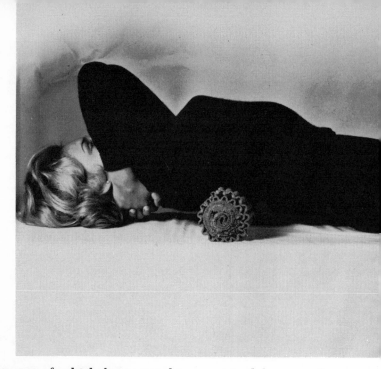

Figure 9

by means of which large weights are raised by use of comparatively small forces.

Since the carpet roll serves the purpose of acting as such a
fulcrum, the respective vertebrae or joint *above* the roll becomes subjected to mild, but scientifically exact applied mechanical force to bring about *speedy re-establishment of normal
joint relationship.* Frequently, distinct snapping or crunching
noises or sensations are felt or heard by the "patient" doing the
exercise.

GENERAL OBSERVATIONS

The lower part of a person's back (lumbar region) is often
under-developed and therefore highly delicate in many individuals. For this reason, it is best to *refrain* at least at the start
with exercising this lower or *small* of our back.

Some of my students have used some additional support
(such as a few books) when they insisted that the whole spine
should be "helped."

At any rate, let us be careful not to cause possible discomfort by using all precautions for weight support in this area, or
confine all exercise to upper back. This means that there are
about six upper vertebraes being helped.

THE HIP MOVEMENTS

There are three phases in this hip corrective exercise. In all movements, the roll is always placed just below the hip (sacrum). To keep body from twisting, both arms are stretched out on floor to provide steady support.

In the first exercise, legs are drawn up to body, feet resting on floor, legs in a vertical position. With legs kept apart about six inches, both knees are now "thrown" forcefully into both directions, left and right. (Figure 10, 11, 12)

In the second movement, the roll is again placed below the hip (sacrum). Both legs are now drawn up to the body with feet off the floor and *rotated in a circular motion clockwise.*

In the third phase, circular motion is directed *counter clockwise.* (Figure 13)

The hip joint, or sacro-iliac articulation frequently becomes twisted out of its normal position. The roll-hip exercises have often helped in the restoration of positional integrity to such involved hip joints.

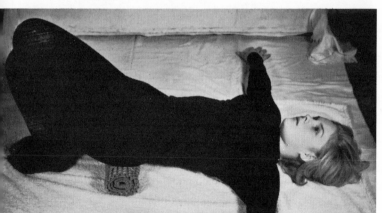

Figure 10

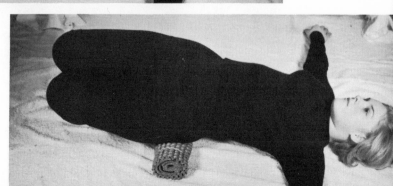

Figure 11

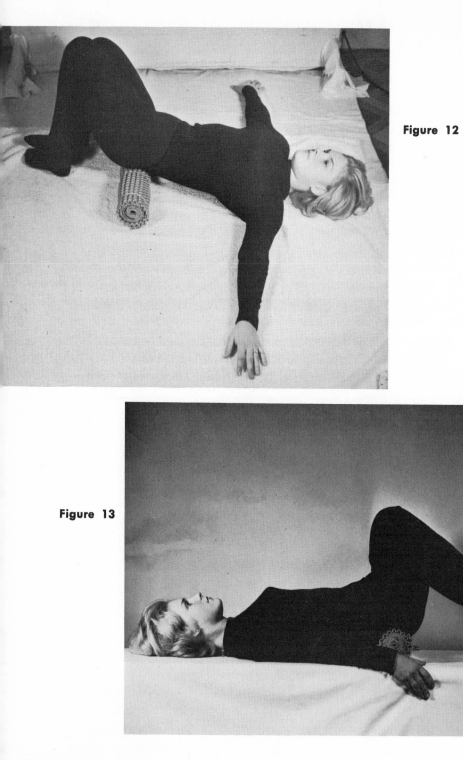

Figure 12

Figure 13

14

HOW TO MAKE THE CARPET ROLL

The basic material is carpet or rug material with some type of sponge rubber covering. Carpet padding, made out of such sponge rubber, works excellently. Any old remnants of rugs or carpets could thus be used. If not on hand, they may be purchased from any carpet or floor covering shop for less than one dollar per roll.

The inner carpet portion measures 18 inches wide by 28 inches long. The outer soft padding material is 18 inches wide (same as carpet) but only 15 inches long (3 inches less than that of width).

It is important to take some effort in "rolling" tightly the carpet into an even roll, with pile portion being on outer side of roll. Follow up by "rolling" around this roll the smaller sponge rubber portion, with rubber side being on outer side of roll.

To make a perfectly tight and even roll, it takes two people or four hands to do the job. The fingers of all four hands are engaged to bend the carpet tightly at the start and roll fabric evenly. A few strong rubber bands stretched over ends of roll will hold it together. The outside rubber padding can then be placed around roll, held firmly in place by more rubber bands, or string.

WHAT IS "NEUROPRACTIC?"

For a number of years I had been engaged as sort of "trouble-shooter." Occasionally, members of the drugless treatment profession would request my services as a consultant in the management of difficult cases.

About eight years ago, I had been called out of state in the case of a young man, suffering serious distortions in neck and hip caused by an auto accident. The patient had been on opiates for a considerable time, but being afraid of addiction, had refused to continue with this treatment. The man was in such constant and agonizing pain that sleep was practically impossible and he was near a state of final nervous collapse.

This case was most pathetic to the attending local doctor

and my collaboration was requested. For years, I had been teaching all sorts of manipulative techniques, used by various members of the drugless profession. Here we could find Chiropractic, Osteopathy, Naprapathy (massage), or any movement observed during extensive searches in all parts of the globe. I had studied methods used by local healers, bonesetters, "heilpracticers," magicians, holy men, fire-walkers, bruchus, etc. The field of observation had been extended to most unorthodox surroundings, deserts or jungle, among the learned and among the primitive.

I had been credited with originating the "Ganglion Impar" treatment, where a specific nerve pressure—application—treatment could afford complete rectal dilatation without the use of anesthesia. I felt I was able to cope with any situation creating human suffering.

The patient was in agony—unable to sleep. My treatment, everything I had learned to bring relief, was without success.

I became frustrated.

What does man do in such a desperate situation? Is it prayer so fervently expressed in the hour of need? It certainly worked, as the occasion developed into this new method of manipulative arts. During the last moments of my attention when it appeared that there was no hope for relief, the patient shouted: "Do it again. Do it again." "What?" I inquired. "Press again on the same spot, the pain there is leaving." What had taken place was the exertion of pressure coming from a pocket knife inadvertently contacting the pain areas during the treatment. The pressure was repeated in affected areas and the incredible took place. *The pain disappeared!* The patient became elated. What a blessing to be free of pain, almost frantic with joy, the patient now could look forward to a speedy recovery.

The new treatment is called Neuropractic, and I have since systematized it in a text book for the manipulative profession of therapy.

Nerve centers and nerve paths are the landmarks for the new pressure applications and specific manipulations bringing about quick re-establishment of nerve conductivity.

In the May, 1961 issue of *The Reader's Digest* appeared the condensation of Kessler's book, *The Man With the Miraculous*

Hands. The book depicts the amazing story of Dr. Felix Kersten, a former masseur, who became a most successful European doctor. In exchange for treatments, the doctor requested and obtained the release of 60,000 victims out of concentration camps and certain death.

I had heard of Kersten's therapy activity before. I never had met the doctor in person, and was anxious to meet the outstanding healer and possibly learn the secret of his success.

I came too late, Kersten had shortly passed away. From those who knew him and from some writings he left behind, an approximate reconstruction of Kersten's method could be made.

An astounding similarity of that with Neuropractic was apparent, as both systems emphasize the correlations of nerves to the rest of the body.

In Neuropractic, the mode of attack is the application of steady pressure, followed by slight massage movements. In this, Kersten only differed by concentrating more on the kneading movement of affected nerve tissues. Neuropractic opens an insight into an amazing behavior relationship between body segments distantly situated.

This phenomenon has been somewhat put to good use in a treating method known as Reflexology. Chief attention in this treatment is usually accorded the soles of the feet, where pressure from the thumb is applied in areas of the sole, corresponding to internal organs having similar nerve supply.

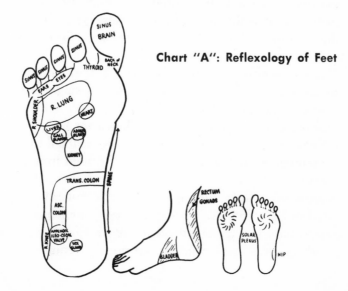

Chart "A": Reflexology of Feet

There is a decided difference in Neuropractic. The lesion, or center of pain is first identified. The searching finger tips quickly can find the right location. The surrounding muscular attachments always are found to be contracted with a characteristic feel of grittiness at the exact region of nerve impairment. Post-mortem examinations have established the nature of this gritty substance, so effectively interfering or blocking the passage of nerve force. The offending material is crystallized uric or carbonic acid, deposited by nature in a shielding mechanism to protect weakened or injured nerve structures. That this helping gesture by nature, so well intended, often has the opposite effect, is a conjecture we need not be concerned with at this time.

The pressure manipulation, starting from the pain areas, follows the course of connecting nerve paths, wherever found to be affected. There are unmistakable signs to the operator, contracted muscles, the "ground glass" feel in nerves. The patient equally knows the operator to be on the right track. There are sharp, cutting pains connected with the treatments. But surprisingly, the pains quickly lessen and more astoundingly, deep seated aches equally shrink. Still more perplexing is the re-orientation of bodily functions, so quickly re-established.

Many times I myself became amazed.

In one case, I treated a doctor having lost his equilibrium and unable to walk unassisted. One hour after a single treatment, the man shouted with joy—he had just completed walking a straight line without outside help. Several such cases reacted in a similar manner.

A boy, age nine, couldn't go to school because of inability to control bowels and bladder. Again, a single treatment restored normalcy.

A nurse, after having been burdened for five years wearing neck collar and lumbar corset had been enabled to discard the equipment, as well as enjoy her first freedom from pain in five years.

Another nurse, suffering from Edema, got rid of her "moon face" fullness and swollen legs in twenty-four hours.

It is only fair to include that the treatments not only consisted of nerve manipulations but equally required the adjustment of bony articulations. The positioning of uppermost segments of the spine, known as Atlas and Axis, are of tremendous significance to the well being of the body.

THE AUTONOMIC NERVOUS SYSTEM

A few important characteristics of the Autonomic Nervous System should be noted. These nerves constitute that branch of the nervous system which controls involuntary functions of muscles, glands and organs. There are two divisions of this regulatory control mechanism. These two divisions are called sympathetic and para-sympathetic chains.

For our purpose it is essential to remember that these two branches are *antagonistic* to each other. One group *exerts increase*—the other, *decrease* in functional capacity.

One group originates in the spine, the other in the skull and lower end of the spine.

It is obvious, that if one group is "strangulated" or obstructed, it can no longer act in a balancing capacity and thus upsets the delicate equilibrium of glands. This may explain the presence of so many systemic disorders so prevalent in the majority of people. Thyroid abnormalities, digestive disorders (stomach, gall bladder, pancreas), kidney or bladder complaints can thus be explained on the basis of disturbance to the autonomic nervous system.

Pertaining to body chemistry, we must conclude that it is the endocrine glands which maintain balancing control. The glands in turn are controlled by the two divisions of this enigmatic nerve supply which are constantly "policing" each other.

If one branch is adversely affected by pressure symptromes, it can no longer exert a controlling restraint to its opposing branch. This explains the phenomenon of Hyper (upper) and Hypo (under) functions of such glands as Thyroid (goiter) or Pancreas (Diabetes).

THE TREATMENT PROCEDURE

Starting to treat a new patient, I pay little attention to taking a case history at the beginning.

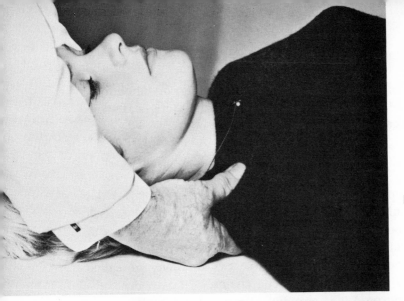

Figure 14

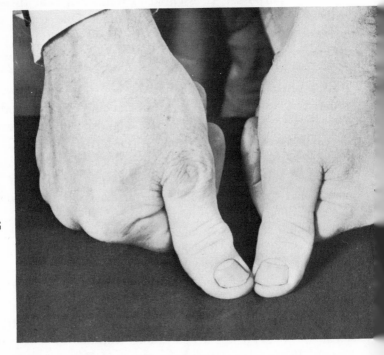

Figure 15

The patient wears a treating gown and lies face up on the table. My first concern is the neck, particularly both sides and below the skull (Figure 14). Figure 15 shows position of thumbs when I check.

Routinely I check all important nerve centers (See Chart No. 1) on front side of body.

What is the "feel," are the tissues rigid or elastic? What is the response of the patient? Do I encounter any painful spots or areas? The facial expression of the patient is a sure guidepost. In this "face up" position I finally come to the feet. A diagnostic feast awaits the examiner. I am not concerned with the soles of the foot in which diagnostic significances have been presented by several authorities. I am mainly interested by the upper portion of the foot which can give many clues as to the condition of the patient.

Chart No. 1

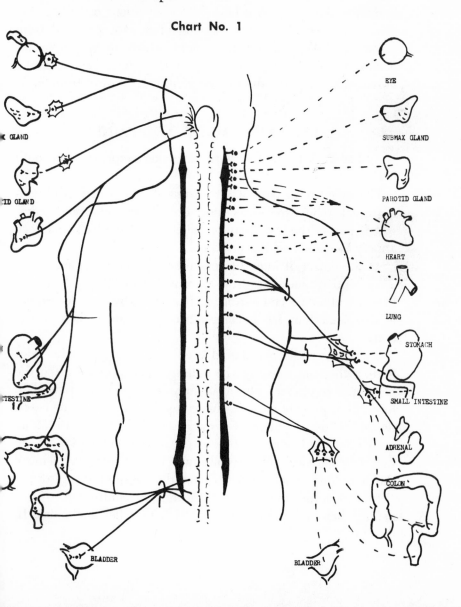

EYE

SUBMAX GLAND

PAROTID GLAND

HEART

LUNG

STOMACH

SMALL INTESTINE

ADRENAL

COLON

BLADDER

The study of the chart will reward the student with more than one solution to a perplexing problem. Not only is one being helped by untying knotty diagnostic problems, but equally benefits by treating these newly discovered "landmarks" with Neuropractic, resulting in the improvement of nerve-distantly-associated body segments.

The patient is then put into a face down position where the most important body components—spine and lateral autonomic chains—are inspected.

How is the spine? Are both fleshy elevations on either side even and free of pain when subjected with pressure from finger tips? How about the sciatic notch to its important Sciatic Nerve? The knee joint is not to be overlooked as nerve impingement may be discovered *before* the start of trouble.

RELIEVING ACHES AND PAINS

And so back to the feet with particular emphasis upon both heels.

The majority of patients are primarily interested in obtaining quick relief from discomfort created by aches and pains.

Any part of the body may be afflicted, but the back and neck appear to command top positions.

At the outset, it must be remembered that aches and pains are essentially messages from various parts of the body to the brain or other nerve control mechanisms. They are to remind us that something has become out of order somewhere in the body.

It is obvious that we should heed such a message—that is of finding the true cause of the aches or pains. Quite often the help of a competent physician may have to be employed to forestall or prevent any possible complication or in some cases, detect the development of a more serious body deterioration.

In other and more gratifying cases, the elimination or removal of the local ache or pain may in itself not only remove the symptoms, but equally correct the cause of the disorder.

In this connection, we are fortunately confronted with a definite behavior pattern associated with aches and pains. If, for instance, we control the ache or pain, we simply observe these cardinal rules:

1. Does the discomfort remain eliminated? or—
2. Does the ache or pain return? And if so, to what degree or intensity?

In the first case, the pain symptrome was of pure local level and possibly caused by some minor irritant or injury, creating nerve irritation. This nerve irritation became intensified by inprecipitation of metabolic end-products, giving rise to a gradual increasing strangulation or blockage of involved nerves. The suggested treatment helped to remove the blockage, thus freeing the nerves from its encroachment with elimination of the aches or pains.

In the second case, the suggested treatment removed wholly or partially all body discomfort but this improvement is only temporary as aches or pains return within a short time, sometimes in an aggravated form.

This state of condition is due to a reflex mechanism instigated from deep seated abnormalities. As formerly pointed out, professional help should be encountered in all such cases, making a complete diagnosis of the systematic involvement with emphasis on correcting the true cause of the disorder.

NORMAL AND ABNORMAL NERVE TISSUE CONDITIONS

Healthy nerve tissue is soft, resilient and elastic. Abnormal nerve tissue is rigid and inelastic.

WHY THE DIFFERENCE IN NERVE TISSUES?

Precipitation of uric or carbonic acid into the covering of nerves is one of the most important reasons. As formerly mentioned, this precipitated material undoubtedly is used by the organism as a protection. It is possible that the affected area had been slightly hurt by having been bruised, squeezed, or injured by other means (chemicals). As a result, the defensive mechanism of the body becomes aroused. The precipitation of hardening or rigidifying material into injured nerves is inaugurated as such, Nature's intent to fortify or protect delicate tissues from the "hostility" of environment and subjected injuries.

So far so good, Nature tried to do the best she could. As fortifying agents it can use only substances available.

Individuals with preponderant protein intake (meat, fish, eggs, etc.) are richly supplied with uric acid. Those of us who partake predominately in carbohydrates, vegetables, fruit, cereals, bakery goods, sweets, etc., may have available generous supplies of carbonic acid.

The insidious aspect of this acid depositing is the process of crystallization. Consistencies of smoothness and elasticity gradually change into hardness and inelasticity, resembling ground glass. Indeed, under the microscope, some of these acid crystals appear like tiny little daggers with razor sharp edges.

Besides acid crystals there could also be deposits of cholesterol (from fat) or calcium carbonate (from perverted bone metabolism or faulty absorption from food).

PAIN SENSATION CAUSED BY PRESSURE

The development of this crystalline material explains the intense sharp pain one experiences by the use of pressure application. How often have I been told to keep my finger nails from digging into the skin of my patients, when in reality only the flat portions of both thumbs had been applied.

RELIEF WITH PRESSURE APPLICATION

The corrective results one can obtain with pressure application is truly amazing. From a mechanical standpoint, we are applying counter irritation with this application of pressure over affected areas. The flat parts of both thumbs are usually used, exerting pressure of from one to as much as fifteen pounds (See Figure 15).

As formerly discussed, an intense pain is felt over "blocked" or "strangulated" areas. This highly acute pain, however, is not constant but is relieved in a relatively short time. In some cases

I have observed the disappearance of pain in as little as five minutes of pressure subjection over a painful region.

COMMON SITES OF PAIN

Any part of the body could become an area of concentrated pain sensation, particularly so, if subjected to injury. These are the cases that respond most speedily to the normalizing effect of pressure application. Pain usually disappears after a single "treatment," but in some persistent cases, applications may have to be repeated several times per week. As to prevalence, the most common pain sites of the body are #1 nerve centers and #2 bony articulations (joints).

NERVE CENTERS

Here we find a more complicated picture. The pain usually is not of local origin but is the result of Reflex action.

It can be taken for granted, that a definite disorder has invaded one or more important organs such as heart, liver, gall bladder, kidneys, stomach, internal glands, etc.

ARTICULATIONS (JOINTS)

The most striking example in this category is found in the 24 segments of the spine. These segments or vertebrae can become out of alignment and thus exert abnormal pressure upon nerve trunks and vessels of circulation that emerge at each spinal joint. In addition, we may consider all other joints such as found in arm, hand, leg, foot, etc. Because of their movability, joints are most vulnerable to become injured and thus form a nucleus for pain concentration.

We can briefly consider nerve tissue to be made out of two parts—that of white matter and that of gray matter. The division in each part is about equal.

Gray matter is that part of the general Nervous System having intelligence to maintain body development and functions as well as possessing the potential for mental and spiritual evolvement.

White matter is devoid of intelligence and is able only to convey messages or impulses from one part of the body to another.

Both gray and white matter, or the entire Nervous System, is involved in becoming irritated by being inprecipitated or strangulated (choked). This is particularly the case when nerve centers have become the target for pain sensations.

NERVE AND MUSCLE RELATIONSHIP

When manipulating nerve centers or nerve trunks, it must be borne in mind that nerve tissues are firmly connected or attached to muscles. For this reason, it could be stated that in reality muscle fibers are being treated, those that firmly surround the affected nerve tissue.

In this connection, a strange relationship exists between muscles and nerves.

Whenever a specific nerve becomes involved with metabolic precipitation, or deposit, its respective functional pattern is immediately retarded, creating a degree of blockage or strangulation in the interpretation or conductivity of nerve energy.

This in turn affects the surrounding muscle fibers by becoming spastic, a degree of rigidity or hardness. In this manner, a chain reaction has been inaugurated with implication of a vicious cycle.

The more obstruction to the nerve—the more rigidity to the muscle, creating still more obstruction to the nerve, and so ad infinitum.

Returning to our first patient, "who inaugurated" Neuropractic, we are reminded that the man had a crushed hip suffered in an accident. The man had been unable to sleep more than five minutes at a time as intense pain in the hip area kept him in agony day and night.

In the frantic attempts of using various types of manipulations, sudden relief had been obtained by an otherwise awkward positioning of the ailing body. Inadvertently, positive pressure had been applied to a specific region, bringing the sudden and mystifying relief of pain. The patient now could sleep uninterruptedly for hours at a time. In a matter of weeks, the patient was back on his feet, able to carry out the work he had been accustomed to.

Another interesting case was that of a man who fell fifty feet into a mine shaft, fracturing hip and 5th lumbar vertebrae. This man had been told that he could never walk again. By virtue of the pressure treatments, he was also returned to

Chart No. 2

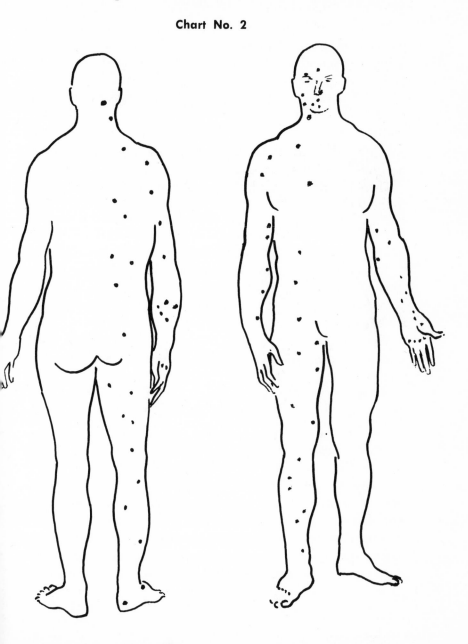

normal life after having suffered agonizing pain for several weeks before receiving treatments.

It is true that often pain does become more intense in an already painful area with the "treatment," but it is also true that such a pain is not seriously objected to by the patient. This is the case whether one treats himself or whether a treatment is given to another person.

The cause of pain is manifold. There could exist a partial paralysis of nerve or muscle fibers with some sensory nerves being over-sensitive. Then, as formerly mentioned, we find the problem of precipitation, uric or carbonic acid in crystallization. The application of pressure into such areas exerts a feeling to the patient as though ground glass is being "rubbed" into their tissues. It is part of the "treatment" to break up or pulverize the deposits for consequent absorption and elimination by the body's functioning.

There could also exist localized inflammation, always painful to the touch.

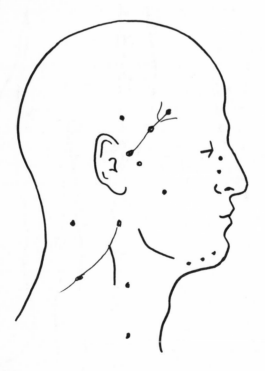

Chart No. 3

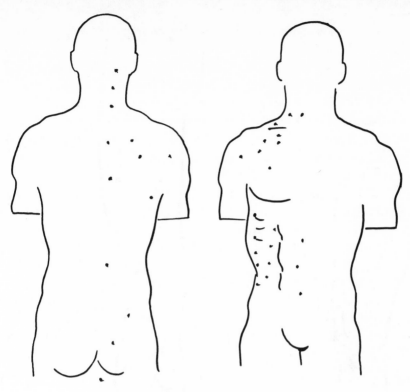

Chart No. 4

AREAS TO BE "TREATED"

As formerly discussed, tissues overlying nerve centers are the most frequent sites requiring attention.

Next in importance come articulations of bones (joints) to be followed by regions of the body subjected to minor injuries (blow, squeeze, effects of chemicals, etc.). The chart of nerve centers will give respective locations of most important pain areas. (Charts 2, 3, 4 and 5)

ABNORMAL HIP (SACRO-ILIAC) CONDITIONS

In this group we find largest percentage of all backache cases.

The disorder is mostly created by some type of physical force such as falling in any direction, forward, backward or sideways. The condition could be caused by any sudden shift

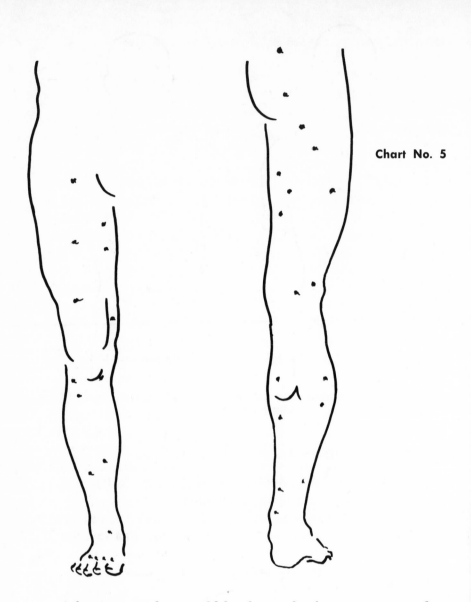

of position such as could be the result of injuries sustained in, or by vehicular accidents.

In other, more puzzling cases, there may exist no apparent reason. Slowly, an occasional sharp pain may develop, gradually changing into a dull ache with greater persistency.

Here, we are confronted with a systemic or constitutional derangement of the nervous system with all the side effects of muscular rigidity—precipitation of acid crystals into involved tissues, etc.

In the majority of cases of hip pains we find a definite mal-position of the joint or articulation. The hip bones (iliacs) have undergone a slight movement from their normal position with the spine (sacrum). In the absence of physical force having caused the positional derangement, what then did cause the change?

The answer lies in the intricate mechanism of the autonomic nervous system with its two branches, one bringing about contraction, the other relaxation. If one of the branches is adversely affected, it can no longer exert balancing action against its opposing branch. Thus, imbalance is the result which, in the case of hip pains could contract the musculature on one side of the hip excessively, while permitting too much relaxation of muscles on the other.

It would take but an insignificant force to "jolt" the joint out of its normal position, such as stepping down harshly from a sidewalk curb or even while sitting in a chair bending side-ways or making a sudden twisting movement. An already established slight irritation to the involved nervous system (caused by now poor protective or surrounding muscle fibers) becomes aggravated, the inevitable course of chain reaction.

Nature also enters the picture by attempting to alleviate pain in the suffering organism. This is carried out by deposit-ing of waste products as fixing agents or protective coverings. The purpose of this precipitation undoubtedly is reduction of motion, as in severe cases occasionally the joint becomes com-pletely immobilized, similar to being "cemented over."

PROCEDURE FOR RELIEF

With both flat portions of thumbs or tips of all fingers operator searches areas of hardness or ropy consistencies, feeling somewhat gritty under finger's touch. The patient will always experience sharp or cutting pain sensation, when af-fected regions are being "discovered." (Figure 16)

Beginning with slight pressure, the operator pushes or presses with both thumbs upon slightly elevated areas. With increasing tolerance of patient, pressure is gradually increased to about fifteen pounds. Stretching of muscles and nerves by

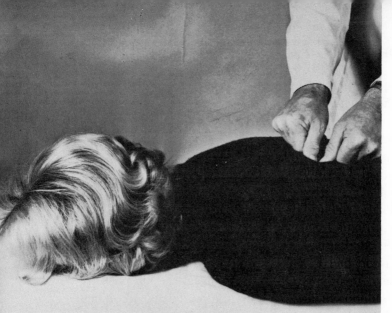

Figure 16

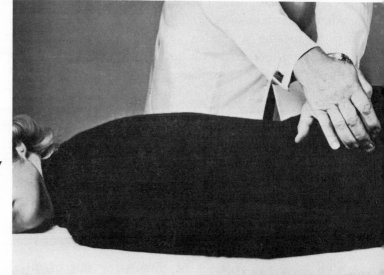

Figure 17

scissor motion is also rewarded with good results. Duration of treatment of single area up to five minutes, entire hip up to one quarter hour. (Figure 17)

With amazing accuracy it will be found that a portion of the pain may have disappeared after the first treatment. In cases of long standing involvement, treatment may have to be repeated every other day for more lasting improvements.

HEART ABNORMALITIES

All heart conditions such as irregular beat, too slow or too fast a beat, flutter, improper valve closure, angina pectoris (clogging of vessels with cholesterol) etc. will show definite signs of nerve blockages in upper left back. (Figure 18 and 18A)

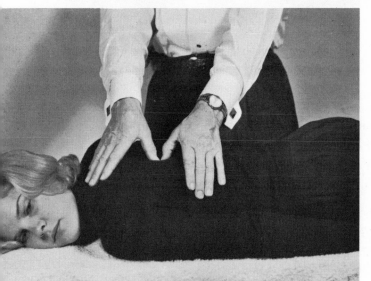

Figure 18

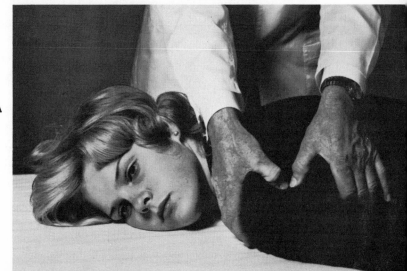

Figure 18A

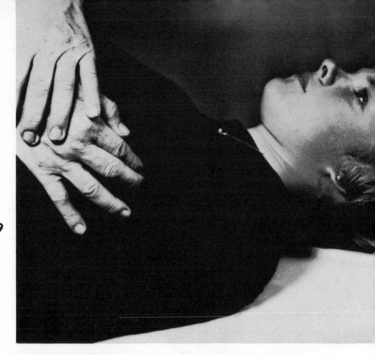

Figure 19

A similar nerve obstruction will be found slightly to the left of left breast nipple.

Use pressure application as outlined above and shown in Figure 19.

TYPICAL BACK ABNORMALITIES

Disc Involvement and Curvatures

This brings up an interesting controversial subject, that of disc abnormalities. We hear of "herniated or ruptured" discs, of misplaced, thinned, squeezed, collapsed or otherwise malpositioned discs.

In my many years of teaching experience, I have never encountered a single case of disc abnormality that could not be helped by Neuropractic. In practically every case, it was found that certain muscle fibers on either side of the spine had assumed contracted or "spastic" inconsistencies with resulting abnormal pull or squeeze to respective spinal region. Thus, one or more discs become subjected to a "lopsided" squeeze, bringing about herniation.

34

Since muscle tonicity is regulated by nerves, it explains the amazing re-orientation or correction of disc abnormalities, when Neuropractic attention is given to the spine as a whole. With patient in face down position, the operator subjects entire back to a visual scrutiny. To what extent does there exist equality in the respective bulgings of muscle groups of one side of the spine in comparison to the other side?

Frequently, one or several areas of abnormal bulgings can thus be discovered.

This easily detectable bulging is the result of local spasticity, created in turn by some type of blocking or strangulating interference to the involved nerves.

Metabolic by-products become attracted to these irritated nerves, resulting in a chain reaction or viscous cycle. In due time the functional ability of the nerve is reduced.

There we find a drastic reduction in the interpretation (gray matter, intelligence) and conductivity of nerve energy (white matter, fibers, conductivity).

So far we have discussed primarily implications affecting the spine. Since we are concerned with nerve and muscle behavior which maintains the very integrity of the spine, we must necessarily delve deeper into the intricacies of the Nervous System.

The Autonomic branch now becomes the target for our investigations. We have learned that this involuntary division is made into two portions, the Sympathetic and para-Sympathetic group. Being *antagonistic* to each other, they either increase or decrease specific functions regulating body chemistry.

Now we are coming to an important positional implication. While there exists but one spinal column, we find *two* distinct autonomic chains situated and running parallel to the spine on either side about midway between spine and outer margin of the back.

Let us now return to a hypothetical case of disc abnormalities. When bulgings of muscles are apprehended, they are found predominantly on *one* side of the spine, indicating interference to nerve control to that specific region. By pressure application as well as various stretching manipulations all spasticities assume lesser involvement. The once hard, rigid, ropy and often gritty characteristic of tissues become soft, pliable and elastic. Most importantly, the patient is amazed and gratified as most acute pain sensations have disappeared (Figure 20 and 21).

A Case History of "Ruptured Disc"

A girl dancer, age 21, suffered from excruciating pain in lower back. It was diagnosed as ruptured disc, as well as lateral curvature of spine.

Examination revealed extreme contraction of right side of back, specifically emphasized in lower back.

The young lady had been the patient of a Chiropractor who had treated the patient for several months. The girl had been afforded partial relief from pain by the Chiropractic treatments but no improvement to the curvature or affected disc. The Chiropractic doctor finally advised the girl to submit to spinal surgery as there was no other way he could suggest in the treatment of this "ruptured disc."

The patient came to my attention during one of my professional classes. At the outset I pointed out the extreme one-sided contraction of back. I pointed to the spine, bent sideways like a bow.

In my commentary on origin and prognosis of condition, I called specific attention to the curvature and its implication to body length. The young dancer, slightly short of stature, was extremely sensitive about her height. I remarked that the girl could be made taller by a few Neuropractic treatments. For the purpose of proving this height increase, I had one of the doctor-students place the girl against the wall to record exact height dimensions. They were told to make a mental picture of the involved curvature.

The ensuing treatment consisted of pressure application of about 10 to 15 pounds, plus stretching deep massage movements to the entire spastic side of back. This treatment, lasting about 30 minutes, gradually softened the "hardened" muscles with most pain sensations disappearing.

The progressive release of abnormal muscle tension permitted the spine to straighten discernibly. The attending student

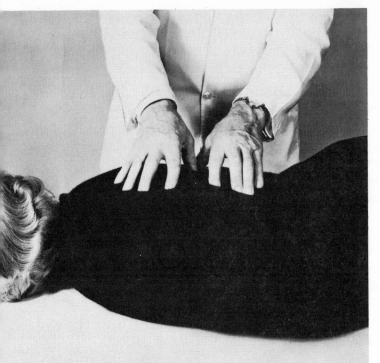

Figure 20

Figure 21

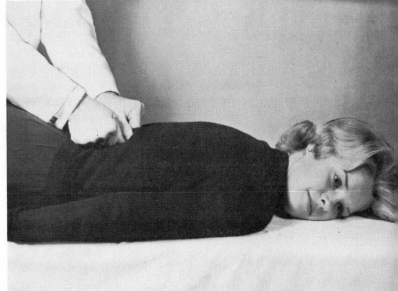

body was amazed to observe the improvement literally under their eyes. Still more dramatic was the rechecking of body height where an increase of *over one inch* had been noted.

The young lady nearly cried for joy, as subjectively she felt the improvement immediately in the relief of pain.

Objectively, the specific and exaggerated bulging on the side of one vertebrae disappeared, denoting the direct release of squeezing action to bodies of vertebraes and permitting disc to assume once more the normal position.

As a follow-up, the patient received two more treatments after which she was discharged as corrected.

It is said that a single swallow does not make a summer and that therefore the outcome of this particular case does not necessarily point to a regular pattern in the disposition of related cases.

In my experience, the only difference I have observed is found in age and history implications of patient.

A definite rule does exist. The younger the patient, the quicker results. Further, if the abnormal condition is caused by external forces (injuries), results are speedier and more positive. Conversely, an inherited physical disorder must be viewed with caution, but often rewarding both doctor and patient with gratifying results.

OTHER SUCCESSES ACHIEVED WITH NEUROPRACTIC

A prominent ball player had been incapacitated from an injury sustained to one of his shoulders. He could no longer "throw" the ball and the club lost one of its "drawing cards." There was little hope that the young man could have put his shoulder into workable condition in order for him to return to his beloved game.

The man received three treatments after which he was discharged. Just a few days ago I saw the notice in the paper where this particular player is back in the harness and apparently fulfilling the high expectations of the ball playing world.

The trainer of one of the big league clubs, having had a thorough training in Physio-therapy, obtained one of my Professional training manuals. Using the book as a guide, he began to employ some of the suggested manipulations and astounded not only himself but equally the club members who benefitted from the new treatment orientation.

In my teaching career, I am reminded about many outstanding improvements Neuropractic was able to bring about.

My regular classes number usually between forty and two-hundred students. The largest class had been comprised of three-hundred and fifty doctors.

The doctor students are requested to bring their difficult or problem cases as treating subjects during class instructions. It can be surmised that over a period of nearly two decades an interesting collection of unusual cases had been appropriated.

Many times the perplexing cases were those of doctors themselves who had been hither and yon to find a solution to their own problems.

Loss of Equilibrium

In one of my classes, a Chiropractor was encountered suffering from loss of equilibrium. The man was unable to walk unassisted and had to be held on either side to keep from falling to the floor.

In the Minneapolis class this man received a single treatment which from all appearances enabled the man to walk without help.

I have had several similar cases where loss of equilibrium was the dominant complaint. Not every case responded as favorably as the one in Minneapolis. But all cases insisted that they had been helped to great extents.

Aggravated Spinal Neck Damage

In my Los Angeles class the treatment was given to a former Colonel of the Air Force. The man had been shot down twice in World War II and suffered from a broken neck, and other spinal damage. Nearly twenty years after the mishap he was still suffering excruciating pains in neck, spine and hip and was unable to walk in a straight manner. The Colonel received two treatments and in his own words he would never be able to thank me enough.

"Frozen" Knees

In my St. Louis class I was asked to treat a Chiropractor who had been unable to bend his legs at the knees for more than *eighteen years*. The man received one treatment of Neuropractic and all of the fifty doctors attending the class instructions at the Chiropractic College auditorium were mystified about the outcome. The *single treatment* resulted in the doctor being able to use his legs in *normal fashion*. He could now sit down in a chair without having to "fall in" as he had been forced to do before.

Head Injury

In my Ohio class, one of the Chiropractors had suffered a head-on collision with his opponent, playing hand ball. The doctor also suffered from loss of equilibrium as a result of which he could practice but one hour daily under the constant guidance of a nurse. The condition had been effective for several years and my help was requested. The doctor received three treatments; from all appearances he was completely relieved of all of his nerve involvements.

Injuries to Infants

In Detroit, Michigan I am reminded about another striking example of what can be attained with Neuropractic. An infant, aged thirty days, was brought to the class in a bassinet. The child, a niece of an attending Chiropractor, had been diagnosed to be a spastic case and told there was no known cure for it. This was my youngest patient, barely weighing twelve pounds. The parents had been told that the child would have to wear steel supports for twelve or so years during the period of most intense physical development.

This was a most puzzling case, the child having been normally delivered without instruments. A single treatment was given in front of the attending class with both parents standing by. After the manipulation, the parents were told to return the following day for our second session of class instructions. There, electrifying results were noted in this child. The head, which had been grotesquely held to one side, was found to be in a normal position. Both legs formerly contortioned almost ninety degrees, were also found to be perfectly straight. The gratified parents were told that there was no need for further attention. Every attending doctor plus myself had been more than amazed about the rapidity of improvement. One of the attending members of the class made the significant statement that Neuropractic, the manipulation of nerve tissue, was as important to the healing profession, as is the self starter to the automobile.

As a general comment, I wish to add that certain bone-setting practices had also been found necessary to be included.

Orifical Techniques

Last but not least, there are certain manipulative techniques referred to as orifical treatments. The oral cavity, the rectum and the female reproductive organs are involved. The Ganglion Impar technique, which affords complete rectal dilatation without the use of anesthetics, is one of the treatments. It must be remembered that at the end of the spine, situated between internal and external sphincter, is a net-work of nerves known as the Ganglion Impar. This pelvic control mechanism is the most important nerve center in the body, outside of the brain. Implication of strangulation or acid crystal precipitation often creates obstructions in this important nerve center, interfering with the maintenance of proper body chemistry. The Ganglion Impar technique not only brings about dilatation of the orifice to its normalcy, but equally affords nerve conductivities to become re-established.

In the female pelvic orifice there could exist all sorts of abnormal conditions. A specific soft tissue manipulation has often resulted in discernible improvements.

For those of my readers who wish to delve deeper into these subjects, the professional treating manual on Neuropractic may be obtained.

DEEP SOFT TISSUE MANIPULATION FORMERLY KNOWN AS "BLOODLESS SURGERY"

Cause of Adhesions

Adhesions are formed as the result of surgery, injuries and after-effects of inflammations. For a clearer understanding, we must study the phenomenon of blood, or serum, clotting mechanism. As is generally known, blood undergoes the process of clotting when it is permitted to escape from its normal confines (that is, vessels). This is essentially a display of body protection, for without this change from a liquid into solids, we would quickly bleed to death in case of injuries.

The same principle also holds true in serum which in composition is identical with that of blood except that it does not contain red blood cells. For this reason the color of serum is amber or straw-like and is clear. If the white of an egg is submerged into boiling water, a significant change in the physical properties of the egg white is noticed. The egg white is no longer liquid but has coagulated into solids. This process closely resembles the clotting of the blood and is of body-protective significance as discussed above.

After the serum has changed into a tough and hardened consistency, another change is discernible, that of constriction. The sticky and plastic material becomes harder and tougher and gradually begins to shrink.

This explains the formation of adhesions. Primarily the serum has oozed out of its confines as result of trauma (injury) or mechanical severance (surgery) or as the result of external forces, due to falls, blows, pinchings, etc. In a large percentage of cases the serum was permitted to escape from its normal confines, because of acute or chronic irritations or inflammations. This is usually observed along the tract of the large intestine, at the border of the pancreas, particularly at the junction of the pancreatic duct with the gall bladder duct (common bile duct). Adhesions are frequently discernible in splenic flexure where they give rise to pseudo heart conditions. Of particular significance, as a result of adhesions, gas accumulations are formed in small pelvis. Female disorders or prostatic involvements are frequently the result of this encroachment of tissue strangulation.

The small pelvis is also often made a target of adhesion production. In the female organism this is often discernible along the tract of both ovarian tubes. Also the uterus itself is frequently involved, giving rise to various abnormal positions of this organ.

The descending colon sometimes is affected in bringing about distortions and anatomical positions in this area, thereby causing all sorts of disturbed functions.

In the male, the prostate gland is often involved with the production of adhesions, giving rise to frequent urination and other male disorders.

The complexities of constipation and intestinal putrefaction (toxemia), undoubtedly are closely geared to mechanical strangulations as are exerted by adhesions. Here we find the formation of pockets (diverticuli), causing stagnation in the passage of feces (stool) with its chain of bacterial multiplication and its production of toxins. In the liver area, adhesions cause stagnation in the flow of bile, and a similar effect is observed along the pancreatic duct where the digestive juice is no longer permitted to flow unimpaired. This gives rise to the traditional complaints of gas discomforts, belchings and bloatings.

DETECTING AND HANDLING ADHESIONS

The discernment of adhesions by finger palpation requires a certain amount of practice. In severe cases, the existence of adhesions can easily be felt under the exploring fingers of both hands. It is essential that the patient is completely relaxed, lying on his back with both legs drawn up.

POSITION OF HANDS

Both hands are employed to produce a scissors effect. All five fingers of the left hand are used to bring about complete immobilization of treated parts. It is essential, that nails are

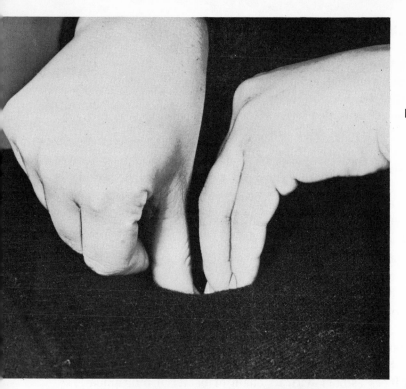

Figure 22

Figure 23

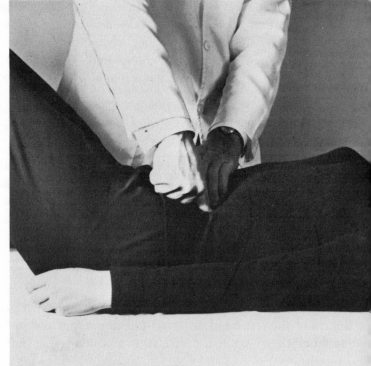

clipped as short as possible and that pressure of finger tips is concentrated on fleshy portion of tips. Deep pressure is exerted in some instances from ten to as much as twenty pounds, to thoroughly maintain immobilization. Pressure is directed downward and somewhat sidewards, this is, toward body of operator. Right hand employs thumb only. That is what I call the "cutting" finger, the "scalpel," or "knife." Again the fleshy or blunt part of the thumb is used in close proximity to fingers of left hand. Actually, the thumb slides along outer border of left fingers, similar to a scissors motion. Pressure is directed straight downward (Figure 22).

In due course the operator will feel a certain "give" or tearing of fibrous bands, resulting in discernible lessening of tension in treated parts. In some instances, former bands, fibers, knots or network of spider-web adhesions can no longer be felt, tissues now feel smooth, straight and orderly. With the tactile finger tips of both hands, the operator now investigates further, and if adhesions are discovered, continues to proceed as discussed above. (Figure 23)

GREAT CAUTION MUST BE OBSERVED

The treatment of all adhesions is comparatively safe and harmless, except wherever there may exist internal ulcers that might break open and produce internal hemorrhages. For this reason, I have always endeavored to impress upon my students to be careful about this one thing: If severe manifestations of pain are observed by the patient during the process of examination, (finger palpation) do not treat directly over the point of pain. In some instances, the fingers can feel strong beats of pulsation due to regional congestion. Stay away from this area. It is surprising to find how speedily improvements are noticed in this region, after a period of three to five days, in which case the detachment of adhesions can be carried a little closer to the critical spot. Obviously this caution must also extend to possibilities of cancer, and an iron-clad rule is to never treat or apply pressure in any way, shape or form to suspected cancer formation anywhere in the body. Follow this cardinal rule and employ professional advice in such cases of severe body disorientation.

DEEP SOFT TISSUE MANIPULATION

Self-Treatment of Adhesions

Patient lies on back with both legs drawn up. With all five fingers of left hand abdominal region is deeply manipulated in the search of tight bands or other constrictive involvements. With flat part of right thumb, assume position of left hand firmly pressing downward and outward to a slight degree. Remember that adhesive tissues are inelastic and will "give" by the pressure of right thumb thus releasing its hold to affected tissues. (Figure 24)

The presence of pockets or diverticulies are the direct results from adhesions. After one area is released from its adhesive grip, proceed to another region and continue until all abdominal tissues assume elastic consistencies.

In this connection it is important to note that adhesions that had been formed as a result of operations, have developed to such strong proportions that they cannot be removed by this manipulative technique. However, so-called spider web adhesions resulting from blow, injuries or inflammations do respond to this treatment.

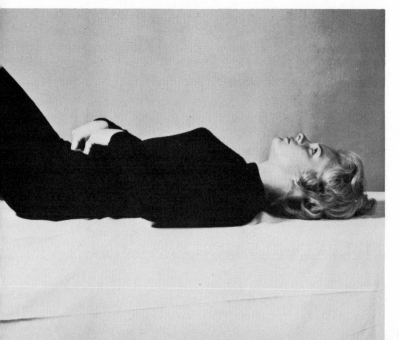

Figure 24

THE NEW DISEASE: "HYPOGENESIS"

Alarming revelations come from Europe about a new disorder afflicting millions and having serious effects. Hypogenesis is relative muscular inactivity. It is most prevalent among persons with sedentary occupations. At less than fifty years of age these people find strong physical exertions difficult.

What had been an everyday muscular load, at an earlier age, has now become an unbearable burden.

The striped muscles make up the main mass of the human body. They exert a direct or indirect influence on blood circulation, metabolism and glandular activities (hormone production). The shape and development of bones are influenced by muscles.

All varieties of action which people take—including mental work—result in muscular movement. Whether a child laughs at the sight of a toy, or a young girl trembles at the first thought of love, or Newton evolves laws of the Universe and writes them down—in every case a muscular movement is a definite fact.

The respective condition of muscles is dependent upon *activity*, muscular *inactivity* is destructive.

In an experiment, twenty-five healthy men between twenty and thirty were confined to bed in a horizontal position for twenty days. They could not sit up, stand up or do any physical exercise. Another similar group were kept in the same condition —except that they performed special exercises four times daily, while lying down.

Within three to five days all members of the motionless group developed back pains, poor appetite and constipation. When they got up after twenty days, they suffered dizziness, blackouts and marked muscle weakness. Their blood circulation was reduced, less blood flowed into their hearts. Their pulse beat rapidly, but the amount of blood pumped by the heart dropped. Sometimes the fast pulse would rapidly slow down, blood pressure would fall and the men would faint.

Here we find typical displays of Hypogenesis. The heart

beats less, lungs breathe less with reduced consumption of oxygen.

The control group, who regularly performed physical exercises in bed during the twenty day test period, maintained their normal physical working capacity.

Prevention of Hypogenesis

How can we prevent Hypogenesis to ourselves? The answer is simple: Let us keep moving, Life is Action. The old adage assumes new proportions: "If we don't use them, we lose them." Muscles with implications to conditioning glands, nerves and organs must be kept in use. Their inactivity results in the breakdown of Metabolism, life slows down and may often come to an end.

Exercise becomes the watch-word. Let us again experience the joy of walking with a little running in between. Household chores should again become playful pleasantries. Let us not forget to work the good soil with its double reward in muscle play and golden harvest.

Muscular activity, every day, should become as indispensable in human life as sleep and food. Daily exercise raises a person's resistance to fatigue. It helps to prevent illness. It increases a human being's life span and years of activity.

ARTIFICIAL FEVER

Give me the ability to create fever and I can cure every disease.   PARMENIDES

The Schlenz Cure

The Schlenz cure derived its name from Mrs. Maria Schlenz who became famous in treating patients with the method of inducing artificial fever by means of over-heated, full baths.

In the Schlenz bath the water temperature starts with that of the body. Hot water is added gradually, thus creating *artificial fever*. One significant contribution of Mrs. Schlenz's discovery is the fact that not only the body but also the head has to be immersed in the tub with only the eyes, nose and mouth extruding. This important rule will prevent any possibility of faintness, caused by over-flooding of the brain with blood.

A similar caution is exercised by the Japanese, who adhere with fanatical regularity to their over-heated baths and who always submit their heads first into the hot water as precaution against faintness.

As stated above, the water has to be equal or slightly above that of existing body temperature. As one becomes accustomed to the heat, hot water is gradually added as a result of which in most cases perspiration will be induced within 20 to 30 minutes. The average duration of the bath is approximately one hour, varying from ¾ to 1½ hours, the patient lying horizontally in the tub with head immersed except nose, mouth and eyes barely above the water line. If the tub is not large enough to accommodate the full length of the body, have legs folded.

After the immersion when profuse perspiration has been induced, the patient is taken out of the bath and wrapped in cotton blankets and then put to bed for another hour or two to finish the period of perspiration.

It has been found that a temperature increase from 2 to 4 degrees F. is sufficient to bring about beneficial effects in the patient. The use of a thermometer would be indicated, but is somewhat difficult to be used by untrained personnel. We can resort to the pulse or heart beat which speeds up in a perfect ratio to internal temperature increase. This ratio is about ten heart beats increase being equal to one degree of fever.

It is best to check the normal pulse rate by placing finger on wrist (radial artery) or neck (jugular artery) and with the second hand of the watch determine its beat per minute. The average count is 72 for male, 80 for female. The normal pulse rate is ascertained *before* the start of the bath. As temperature increases, the pulse rate speeds up and can be checked conveniently at intervals. If, in the case of a female patient, the pulse rate was eighty at the beginning and has now advanced to 110 beats per minute, an increase of 30 beats would indicate a fever of 3.0 degrees. Adding this 3.0 fever to normal body temperature of 98.6 would give us an elevated temperature of 101.6 which is decidedly effective and safe.

Sauna Baths

In my study of contemporary living patterns throughout various parts of the world, I am strongly reminded about the Sauna bath of the Finnish people. The principle of the Sauna bath is subjection to steam-saturated, over-heated rooms where equally the body is responding by developing increased temperatures. Doesn't this remind us of what we have been discussing? We could no more expect these hardy and vigorous people of the European North to do without their Sauna baths at regular and precise intervals than we could expect the American people to do without food. A healthy and deeply ingrained custom has proven over generations the wisdom of a specific way to preserve or regain health. The emphasis, however, in this case is placed on preservation as verified by the enviable vitality of these sturdy people.

Schlenz Bath Effectiveness

The Schlenz bath can be made still more effective by having the patient wrapped in a wet sheet after coming out of the tub. The sheet then is covered with a plastic material or oil cloth which serves a double purpose in preventing the moisture from penetrating into the bed, as well as prolonging the increased temperatures inside the body.

This treatment is possibly the most efficient means of correcting deep-seated and stubborn types of degeneration second only to fasting.

The European experts strongly suspect a *hormone* or *healing like substance being created by the body during the fever period*. It is claimed that it is this substance which is accountable for the many astounding recoveries recorded. No wonder, this procedure, in Germany, has been called the treatment for incurable diseases.

It is important for us to remember that fasting and fever do not go together. The remedy is somewhat weakening and should not be repeated oftener than five to seven days.

2

Conditioning the Body
Permanently for Beauty and Health

ISOMETRIC CONTRACTION

In the past few years the isometric principle in exercising has been tested and approved by the top athletes of the country. Starting as a military secret, this system of no pain— no sweat—muscle building is an equally worthwhile technique

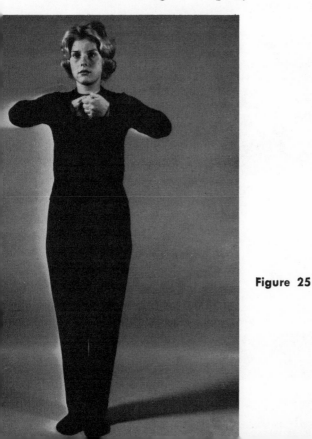

Figure 25

for ordinary men and women who have little time for regular exercises.

The term isometric means "equal measure" which is exactly the amount of contractile force expended by opposing body members.

Figure 25 indicates such a movement. Both arms are raised to nearly horizontal level; interlock both hands and try to pull apart by contracting muscles in arms and shoulders. Hold contraction up to the count of six and relax. The opposite exercise is to push with both arms against hands. Again hold contraction for six counts. Repeat these two movements three times while practicing *deep breathing*.

The fair sex will particularly notice improvements in breasts and neckline.

HOW TO GET SHAPELY LEGS AND THIGHS

Lie on floor and with ankles press against legs of chair (Figure 26). In second movement, place feet inside of legs and press outward (Figure 27).

Figure 26

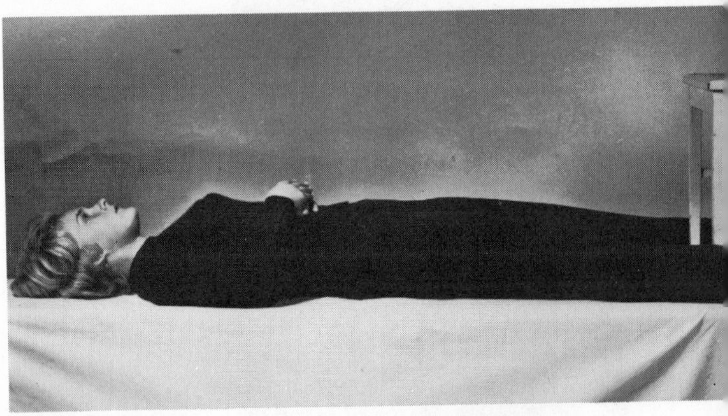

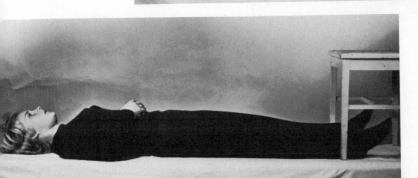

Figure 27

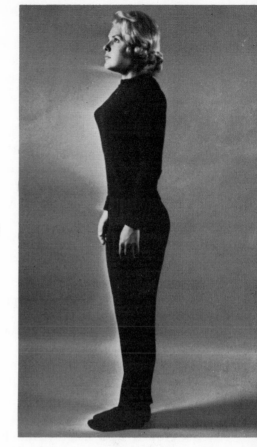

Figure 28

QUICK SLIMMING OF WAISTLINE

Stand straight with arms hanging loosely. Contract abdominal musculature and attempt to draw up stomach as high as possible (Figure 28).

It is important to remember that all of these isometric contractions are to be held for a period of six counts or seconds and then relax. The movements are usually repeated three times accompanied by deep, rhythmic breathing. It is said that if only ten minutes per day are spent with these contractions, muscles can be greatly strengthened, resulting in more buoyancy and well being.

It is up to us to use our ingenuity and think of various positioning to bring into play muscles in need of toning up.

While sitting on a chair, one could hold with both hands on

side of chair. First movement would be to contract arms and back, and pull down. The opposing movement attempts to push up with arms, while resisting with back.

To more specifically firm neckline, clasp hands and place behind nape of neck. With arms attempt to pull head forward, while head is resisting. The side way movement consists of placing right hand against right cheek attempting to push head toward the left, with head resisting pushing toward right. The same movement is carried out on left side, always holding contraction for six counts and repeating three times.

There are innumerable ways in which isometric contractions can be employed. Use your own imagination, spend ten minutes per day and watch results.

DO NOT FORGET THE SUN

The sun is the great source of all power, organic or inorganic, on this planet. Sunlight is essential to all animal life and the higher plants for the processes of assimilating the elements of soil and atmosphere. Especially needed are the ultra-violet rays for the production of the electro-chemical effects.

The human body is directly dependent on sunlight for its growth and healthy development. Deficiencies of sunlight bring on reduction of red blood cells, inducing leukemia, a sickness denoting great increase in the number of white cells. A total exclusion of sunlight may induce severe forms of anemia.

Frequent exposure of the naked body to sunlight will assist the organism in the performance of all functional activities. Sunlight is the best germicide, but could destroy body cells. Moderation should be exercised.

At the start, fifteen to twenty minutes is enough. The rays of the morning sun are particularly beneficial.

Dr. Rollier of Switzerland, treated deformities of children and adults with no means other than sunlight and diet. Permanent corrections were achieved.

Any skin condition, itching or scaling will speedily adjust itself to the healing rays of the sun.

THE ELECTRICAL PHENOMENON OF LIFE

The human body is both motor and generator of electrical energy. In this respect we are somewhat similar to the electric eel, only differing in the respective power release. The electric eel's energy potential is decidedly less than that of man but the release mechanism in the acquatic organism is much more sudden if not "explosive." The electrical charge is strong enough to kill a full size man.

In the human organism, the electrical potential has certain slumbering traits, which, if released at once would only be strong enough to create a glow in a light bulb. Yet, this electric force in the human body is intrinsically more powerful, even though in a latent form, than that of the eel. This electric quality has also been termed magnetism. Where and how did this electrical force develop? It is known that our star bound missiles in outer space obtain certain energies from the sun, stored in solar batteries. This same power has been operating on the crude mineral elements of the earth since primeval ages. The result of this solar radiation is ionization. Ions are the stabilizing forces of life.

The ionization process affects minerals such as calcium, phosphorus, magnesium, sodium, etc. These minerals become part of our tissues and fluids, and require to be constantly replenished through the ingested food.

All ionized minerals are divided into positive and negative polarities. The large number of trace elements possess these precisely arranged polarities of positive and negative charges. This explains among other phenomena the mystifying actions of the endocrine glands with their hormone production. Science has made great strides in the awareness and investigations of ionized substances. Through the spectroscope, man has been enabled to identify respective mineral elements making up man, animal or plant. By means of polarized light it is now possible to ascertain the disposition of the ions.

In life, the tissues of man or animal reveal a definite pattern of movement in their ionized make-up. This action is the result of attracting and repelling polarities of negative and positive forces. In death, the polarized light shows no movement in the mineral elements, all opposition or antagonism has come to an end.

From a philosophical angle we may inject the thought about life, that in its most minute form it expresses action, opposition and antagonistic behavior as exemplified in constant battles.

SOURCES OF IONIZED MINERALS

In plant life, the process of ionization is maintained after the harvest of the plant. Plant tissues then are still alive, full of electric potential to be bestowed to man or beast.

A gradual decline of ionic action is discernible in direct ratio to time and condition of storage. Seeds with durable coverings seem to maintain ionic interchange for longest periods, providing their insulating housings are preserved. "Live" grains several thousand years old have been found in Egyptian tombs.

Wilting of fruits and vegetables plus heat slows down the speed of ion transfer until it comes to an end. In cooking, this gradual destruction of ionization is accomplished immediately.

Minerals in sea water show most the active processing of this magnetic behavior. This explains the amazing recuperating force and life principle of sea water.

Synthetic or *refined* natural foods exposed by polarized light, equally indicate lack of ionization or magnetic qualities.

The green carpet of the earth, next to the seas is our primary source of ionized minerals—being alive and able to bestow life. Only through photosynthesis is the electrical life potential imparted.

The impact of natural and uncooked food orientation is focused by this electrical magnetic-ion—life relationship.

3

Aches and Pains
Relieved with the Fast

The time was winter of 1937 when I became acquainted with the Fast.

Acquainted does not succinctly express the relationship I made with the Fast at that time—more appropriately expressed, the Fast saved my life! I always had been a hard worker but equally—a "hard liver." Blessed with a keen appetite, I loved to eat "good sustaining foods" with a persistent partiality toward steaks and sausages.

Before retiring at night, I had usually consulted the refrigerator and selected generous and "delicious" morsels to sustain me through the night.

With undramatic suddenness the inevitable consequences of this extravagant food emphasis made its appearance. A persistently sharp pain radiating down my left arm had been felt for several weeks. All at once, this slight dull pain became excruciatingly sharp and then it happened. In a flash I lost all strength, could neither stand nor sit—I slumped to the floor feeling a terrific pain throughout my upper left chest.

My Death Sentence

My own diagnosis of a heart attack had later been corroborated by a specialist. Yes, so it was stated, a severe case as indicated by both x-ray and electro-cardiograph. The crisp

professional verdict placed little consideration to possible recovery, but stressed the element of time. Of how much time
there was still left to get things in order. Had I made a will or
testament? What about dispositions as to cremation or burial?

The laconic advice of the specialist: I may have several days,
perhaps up to a week or two.

In a couple of days, the organism crept over the first shock.
I could stand up in a slouching manner and with dragging
feet manage to get around slowly.

This happened on a cold January day. Immediately it was
decided to go to Florida to spend the last fling of life in the
sunny South. The hotel facing the beach made it easy for me
to enjoy the warm sun and soothing sand.

Slowly the pain in my chest became less intense but the
general weakness prevailed. While spending most of the day
lying in the sand on the beach, I had noticed a group of young
people playing vigorous games nearby. These people were in
their early 20's and both boys and girls displayed remarkably
well developed bodies.

How I Beat the Death Sentence

One day I was asked if I would like to join in their game.
My answer—gladly would but could not—that I was a very sick
man, feeling decidedly sorry for myself. Then, by all means,
they insisted, I should meet their idol and teacher—Bernarr
MacFadden, who without a doubt, could help me to get well.
To me, this suggestion first appeared fantastic, if not ludicrous.
Had not the diagnosis of my condition been established by
"unquestionable" scientific means? Had I not been convinced
that there was no "cure" for such a discernible Heart crippling
as affected me? On the other hand, my new friends were so
obviously earnest, sincere and convincing. With a Messianic
zeal they practically carried me to that great man, Bernarr
MacFadden, who, I believe, has done more for the benefit of
humanity here in America than any other man in his time.

I was given a tedious "going over" by the great reformer.
In concise language I was told that what I needed was a
thorough "cleaning out" by a prolonged fast and that I should
start immediately. What transpired since, speaks for itself. Not

only was the irrefutable negative prognosis exploded, all formerly learned concepts pertaining to Health and disease had to be subjected to a painful re-evaluation.

I underwent a complete fast for twenty-eight days. Most surprisingly—at the end of this "ordeal" I felt stronger than at any other time. I could run and play now with the other younger set, which they considered "routine" experience.

Since then I have fasted up to fourteen days several times. I always felt like shouting to the entire world about this true panacea of recreating or maintaining genuine pleasures of living.

I have since overseen or conducted fasts on several thousands of patients and students. The beneficial results have always been not only astounding, but unbelievable in some cases. As to condition of the heart, the organ gradually resumed its normal functional pattern. All pains disappeared like magic— up to now—after twenty-eight years.

We shall examine the intricacies of fasting as practiced throughout the world and ages.

Fasting in Ancient Times

Fasting is as old as is life. Nature provided both feast and famine to maintain balanced organisms for all living things. Take away either one, we will find degeneration and ultimate death. The periodic occurrences of droughts, floods, quakes or other destructive manifestations on the surface of this globe could be interpreted as such a control mechanism. Implications of feasting could thus be checked.

It is for this reason perhaps that nearly all religions made ample use of the fast. Christianity made it obligatory for its members to fast fully two days per week—Wednesday and Friday. This fasting adherence had been prevalent from the second to the fourth century.

Throughout the Orient and among many primitive tribes today, fasting periods supersede most magical and psychic initiations.

In the Bible, fasting is frequently mentioned in connection with prayer. Forty day fasts were experienced by Jesus, Moses and Elijah.

Hippocrates, the greatest physician of antiquity, who lived from 460 to 377 *before* Christ, undoubtedly influenced the great religious and philosophical leaders.

Mohammed, Buddha, Confucius and others fasted for the purpose of favoring a condition of visionary illumination.

In ancient Egypt, syphilis was successfully treated by the Fast.

Fasting in Recent Times

In more recent times we find Dr. Tanner, who shocked the scientific world by fasting once forty and a little later forty-two days under strict observation. There were other doctors such as Graham, Shew, Page, Trall, etc., who could see the tremendous implications of the Fast and used it in their treatments.

Dr. Dewey's descriptions of the Fast are literary gems.

Bernarr MacFadden in his *Physical Culture* helped to spread the knowledge about fasting to the general public throughout the world.

In this connection I must confess that at one time I belonged to the group of people who had their minds made up and didn't wish to become confused by facts. This is why it took a nearly fatal impact to teach me the lesson of not condemning anything *before* investigation.

In Europe, particularly Germany, The Fast had made amazingly great progress in medical circles.

Schroth System

However, the actual start of a systematic fasting cure was made by a lay person, the farmer Johann Schroth 1798-1856. Schroth developed a much enlarged and completely stiffened knee as the result of having been kicked by a horse. The farmer had previously observed injured animals refusing all food until cured. Schroth used alternately fasting and application of hot packs which in a short time restored the crippled leg to its full use.

The Schroth Fasting cure became famous and the country of Austria officially maintained a state-supported Schroth Institute. It is interesting to note that, equally, Priessnitz and Father Kneipp, the famous water treatment pioneers, were outside the accepted Healing Profession.

Moeller System

In more recent times, it was Dr. Siegfried Moeller who found the courage to use the Fast in his practice. He himself fasted several times up to twenty-five days. Fasting meant to Moeller an excellent means to "regain possession of Mind and Body faculties."

Moeller fasted often and gladly not only to overcome minor body discomforts, but mainly to compensate for vacations he could not afford to take. As an over-worked physician in a sanatorium his "frequent vacations" consisted of taking short fasts from six to ten days. By this method, Moeller claimed, he could maintain his over exertions in his work despite an inherited weak constitution.

Riedlin System

Dr. Gustav Riedlin is considered the oldest Medical doctor in Europe having used fasting in spite of tremendous medical opposition.

According to Riedlin, living force is not a physical—chemical problem, but essentially mental and spiritual. The human body is not a machine or boiler which could produce Energy by food combustion. "The living force is certainly depended upon the all permeating cosmic energy. This cosmic energy is equally contained in the food itself, particularly in unheated fruits and vegetables."

Riedlin reasoned that if the purpose of food is to replace worn out cells, furnish energy for Mind and Body as well as create warmth, then logically with the increase of food there should be more warmth and energy. This is not true—The opposite effect is noted. By less food and more rest, more strength would accumulate.

For Riedlin Fasting was a natural process, presented by Nature and "only waiting to be acknowledged by man." There were two distinct steps in the Fast—one to obtain physical improvements, the other to reach spiritual awareness.

Kapferer System

Dr. Richard Kapferer should next be regarded as an early medical pioneer to bring fasting into focus of scientific evaluation. As a child, he met the powerfully built Father Kneipp. Ever since, his parents and four brothers always had resorted to occasional short fasts with intermittent fruit days, whenever slight diseases made their inroad.

Kapferer went from Kneipp to Riedlin. Both were first rank healers, both fought heroically for the acceptance of fasting as a most effective therapeutic force. While Kneipp put most emphasis on his Water Cure—and subjected his patients to only short fasts, Kapferer insisted on continuation of the fast until completion of the internal cleansing process.

Kapferer's contribution to the progress the Fast made in being accepted and recognized by the Medical profession, is contained in his precise scientific papers he presented to his colleagues from time to time. This does not mean, however, that the battle was won entirely, for this we shall have to wait a little longer, as we shall see.

Fasting Recognized Generally

Dr. Otto Buchinger undoubtedly is credited with overcoming the last vestiges of opposition among the Medical profession to the Fast. For one, Buchinger had and still has a commanding personality, extremely intelligent and well educated.

As has been the case in practically every Fasting doctor, personal disease experiences drove Buchinger to the Fast. At the age of forty, he had attained the highest position of a Doctor in the German Navy—that of Fleet Surgeon, equal in rank to that of Rear Admiral.

At the time of his appointment to the top position, Buchinger simply became too sick to carry on and was discharged (1917) as totally incapacitated. The disease: Joint arthritis, severe gall bladder and liver disorder. At that stage, Buchinger gave up all hopes of ever getting well and even considered suicide.

A former Navy acquaintance met the suffering Buchinger and suggested he see Riedlin who, "positively" could help. Surprisingly Buchinger consented since everything else had been tried in vain.

Riedlin prescribed a long fast which was rigidly adhered to for nineteen days. Some complications with the liver and gall bladder developed, making it necessary to break the fast. The arthritic condition, however, had been greatly improved. Buchinger now could get around fairly well.

A second fast of thirty days was then undertaken with Moeller at Dresden. After this, a complete correction of all affected organs and limbs resulted.

With his great mind, energy and thankfulness, Buchinger now resolved to "pay his debt" by making the Fast available to the masses, as well as subjecting it to rigid scientific investigations. It is to Buchinger's credit, that today the majority of European physicians no longer scoff or ridicule the fast as "hunger cure" and accord the subject its rightful place in Therapeutics.

Buchinger has control of two large Sanitariums in Germany that up to now have fasted over forty-thousand patients. With characteristic "Teutonic thoroughness," every detail of the fasting process had been explored by a number of experts. The microscope and laboratory played an important part in these investigations of saliva, secretions, urine, feces, pus, etc. Also examined were skin, body weight and facial expression.

The evidence is irrefutable. Fasting, if properly conducted, is not only perfectly safe, but provides the most effective and speediest recovery from nearly all bodily disorders.

Patients are coming from all parts of the world. Even our famous diet authority, Gaylord Hauser, spent two weeks recently to obtain the benefits of temporary food withholding. There are many wealthy people that can be seen at Buchinger's resorts. They, of all people, certainly could afford the most expensive foods. Yet, the complete fast is religiously adhered to.

Average Length of Fast

The average fast takes in about two weeks. In more drastic cases, up to thirty days is considered necessary to bring the internal cleansing and healing process to completion. In some still more advanced cases of organic degeneration, the fast may have to be repeated, to be taken in several stages. Of utmost importance is the breaking of the fast—a much involved dietary problem.

The Meaning of Disease

Before discussing the general attitude of the body to the fast we must first investigate the *meaning of disease*. With the exclusion of all traumatic (injury) cases, we find that in practically all instances the diseased condition of the body is caused by abnormal metabolism, meaning upset in chemical changes continually going on in the cells of living matter. There are many intricacies to this process of metabolism, but for our purpose it suffices to learn that certain cells and tissues throughout the body become targets of waste precipitations.

This waste infusion is the result of abnormal bowel behavior with certain changes of bacteria instigating poison production, which we shall investigate later in this book.

Some of these waste entities undergo drastic chemical changes, such as uric acid, which may assume a crystalline structure. Here we also find carbonic acid, cholesterol, chlorine, calcium carbonate, etc., to create cellular obstructions by the simple reason of their presence. The connective tissues are foremost chosen for this depositism, but this intrusion could equally extend into the very substance of organs or glands. The coverings of nerves become also involved with such precipitation. In most cases the intruding material is uric acid, which, when crystallized exerts the characteristic cutting pain when subjected to pressure.

The German physicians have termed this infused waste material *Zellenschlacken,* literally meaning *cell cinders.* In England, the term *cell carbon* has taken root—meaning the same thing. As can be surmised, the very presence of this encroaching material creates the problem of blockage.

WHAT OSMOSIS MEANS

In this connection we must necessarily digress to consider the intrinsic implications of osmosis. Osmosis is defined as a tendency of fluid substances, separated by a porous membrane, to filter through it and become equally diffused.

We all know that blood carries the nutrition to the cells and in turn brings from the cells waste products to the organs of elimination (lungs, bowels, kidneys, skin). What is not usually known is the fact that blood as such does not make direct contact with the cells except by permeation through a porous membrane.

Since metabolic waste products do invade not only connective tissue but equally vessels of circulation (lymph and blood), nerve tissues, glands and organs, it can be seen that the degree of porosity of membranes of cells or tissues can be greatly reduced.

Cholesterol is one of these metabolic by-products, a sticky and chewing-gum-like material which has a tendency to become deposited within the linings of vessels, particularly that of the heart. The lumen of the vessels thus become reduced. But still greater harm is inflicted to the microscopic hairlike capillaries where even the tiniest amount of coating could interfere with its osmotic principle, that of permitting the passage of fluids through its pores.

Another aspect of retarded osmosis in connection with altered metabolism can be observed with our most important regulators of body chemistry—the endocrine glands. They also are termed ductless glands as their secretions are conveyed to the bloodstream not directly by duct but by osmosis—secretions are permeated through porous membranes into the circulation.

Since all deposited waste products exert a definite degree of blocking to the various porous cell membranes, osmosis is retarded correspondingly. In turn metabolism, or body chemistry, is interfered with, resulting in the break-down of functional capacity.

I do not believe there exists a single disease in which the above described mechanism of defective osmosis is not at least partially responsible for the disorder. In many or most cases, faulty osmosis is the only real cause of the sick organism, as has been proven in numerous cases. Take away the inner clogging, smudge or obstructive matter (Zellenschlacken or cell cinders), and we will find renewed osmotic efficiency bringing about re-established balanced body chemistry.

HOW THE FAST OPERATES

The complete or partial fast will do exactly that of freeing the body from its encroaching precipitations. If food is withheld from the outside, the body immediately begins to feed itself from within. The "inner physician" takes over and wisely relegates the available reserves to be used for sustenance in an order of inverse ratio of need to the organism. What is least essential to the body is used or oxidized first.

In this category we find mucus, fat, diseased cells or tissues, substances causing obstructions. They are *uric acid*. Undoubtedly this is the most destructive agent, particularly in Westernized countries with their emphasis on protein food.

Ragner Berg, the famous European food expert, once called protein that kind of a food which must be *earned*. If ingested beyond body needs, it will leave its residue such as urea, ammonia, etc. within the body tissues. Uric Acid becomes more insidious by undergoing crystallization. These fine, sharp crystals, resembling ground glass, inflltrate most anywhere in the body but have some preference for the lower extremities (gout) as well as coverings of nerves. Heavy meat eaters are prone to become "saturated" in various degrees from this metabolic waste. Next in importance is cholesterol, this smooth substance has an affinity for the inside of vessel walls, particularly that of the heart (coronary circulation). This coating within the fine capillaries can become catastrophic to those endowed with good appetites, as I had to experience in my own case. Cholesterol becomes one of the targets in the selection of combustibles by body intelligence. I have observed several cases of heart involvements (angina pectoris) clear up in less than ten days on a complete Food rest.

Calcium Carbonate

Whenever this hardening or rigidifying substance makes its presence in the body, we can expect cementing effects to be noticeable anywhere. If bones or joints are affected, we speak of arthritis. The infusion into muscles is termed rheumatism. This perverted type of calcium may invade vessels (artherosclerosis) or organs or glands.

The source of calcium carbonate is faulty food assimilation. Glandular abnormalities are the cause for this "twisted" distribution of the calcium molecule. It appears that the calcium is withdrawn from the bones to become re-deposited in the soft tissues.

The Fast will quickly reshuffle the arrangement of mineral components. In cases of arthritis, the affected joints become less painful, with rigidities abating. I have seen stiff hands again move fingers for piano playing in a matter of twelve days. During the fast, the calcium becomes dissolved to serve the body as nutrition—or eliminated. The urine of fasting arthritics frequently show this whitish settlement in specimens collected for examination.

Carbonic Acid

Those of us who have a "sweet tooth" or partake their food generously from starches, (bakery goods, grains, potatoes), may have to consider their aches and pains coming from carbonic acid. Unlike uric acid, this substance has an affinity to muscular tissues giving rise to rheumatism. Carbonic acid also undergoes crystallization which explains the sharpness of rheumatic pains.

The dissolving action of the fast to this substance is somewhat slower than found in cholesterol and calcium carbonate.

Chlorine

There we find an interesting display of body intelligence. Chlorine is derived from sodium chloride—common table salt. The too generous use of table salt has become a controversial issue for many years. Many European diet experts (some of whom are Nobel prize winners) deplore the over-use of salt. It is claimed that soduim chloride does not undergo assimilation and that therefore it disrupts metabolism. Salt is separated in the body to sodium and chlorine. Sodium is used to neutralize acids of those partaking of predominant acid reacting foods (proteins, fats, starches, with little fruits or vegetables, having alkaline reaction). The leftover chlorine is stored in the connective tissues, particularly having an affinity directly below the skin. The thin, shiny (cigarette paper) skin in hands or feet of the aged is a classical sign of chlorine deposits below. It is one of the gratifying signs of a faster to watch the gradual change in the skin appearance. Even those of advanced age observe a slow but persistent approach of velvetness with finer texture appearing in their skin.

Alkaloids and Drugs

These entities also are to be eliminated by the body although greatly taxing the faculties of both doctor and patient. The drug Theobromine, as contained in coffee, tea or cocoa is cumulative in parts which have not been eliminated. In the network of the connective tissues these retained particles are "stored" possibly "coated or encapsuled" to permit maintaining a passive behaviour.

The Fast now first tears down the insulating coverings to get at the invader. A similar procedure is carried on with other drugs such as pain or sleeping pills or tranquilizers.

The faster, all of a sudden, may experience severe reaction affecting his Nervous System. In several instances, I had to have the patient interrupt the fast, to be carefully concluded in several repeated stages. Often, such cases presented muscular rigidities and spasms resembling epileptic seizures.

But the Fast does come to the rescue and final victory. As the great Buchinger said: "When you subject yourself to a Fast, you have at your command the services of two thousand of the best trained surgeons, who cannot make a mistake, because they are under divine guidance."

CLARIFICATION OF TERMS AND MEANINGS

There exists some ambiguity or misunderstanding in some of the Fasting literature. The words Toxemia, Toxicity, poisons, or poisons in the blood are frequently used.

The Orthodoxly trained physician becomes somewhat reserved with this terminology, even though he cannot refute the over all implication of the presented thoughts.

Toxic means poisonous and the blood stream of even the sickest is rarely poisonous. My observations in dissections and post-mortems conveyed to me that the blood as such has little actual content of demonstrable poisons. There are only about six quarts of blood, constantly changing according to conditions of bowels, liver, bone marrow, etc. Of course this does not mean that the blood does not become "diseased" also. But such disorders should be considered as symptoms of the entire deranged human structure. Anemia, as an example, could be construed as having its origin not in the blood but in faulty liver and bone marrow condition, resulting from abnormal metabolism. Nutritional deficiencies also could upset the mineral or hemoglobin relationship.

"CELL CINDERS" AS CAUSES OF DISEASES

The European terminology of "cell cinders" as cause of disease most accurately drives home the point. It is generally agreed that civilized eating practices make all of us prone to over-eat. It is said that up to the age of twenty, man can eat as much as he can—up to forty as much as desired and after that he should eat as little as possible. Hippocrates made the statement that "if a sick person is fed—one feeds the disease. On the other hand, if the sufferer is withheld from food the disease is fasted out." How true, as I have observed in thousands of cases.

The disease process begins most gradual but insidiously. In metabolism we find two stages, one of building up—the other of tearing down. The latter stage is the guilty one. Foods are not completely torn down and eliminated as formerly mentioned. Uric and Carbonic acid remnants may undergo crystallization, obstructing metabolism. Cholesterol may clog lining of vessels and capillaries, where in some cases it may create starvation in the midst of plenty. Calcium carbonate may infuse joints, muscles or vessel structures, bringing on arthritis, rheumatism or hardening of vessels.

THE "TOWEL-SALT WATER" EXPERIMENT

For best illustration, let us take a small towel. Let us dip this fabric into a solution of salt water. The towel is permitted to dry after which we will find a drastic change in the appearance and "feel" of the material. No longer does the towel feel soft and pliable—it is now rigid like a board and feels hard and brittle. In the immersion, the salt water saturated through the fabric as a liquid but in the drying process changed into crystals. On closer examination we would find the crystals over, under and around every fiber.

Such is the case as so pointedly termed "cinder infusion" by the European experts as bringing on the ravages of disease.

SECONDARY CHANGES THAT HAPPEN

It is axiomatic that *Secondary* changes usually occur as the result of this cell strangulation. Tissues, organs or glands become diseased and undergo degeneration. Necrosis, (tissue destruction) is frequently observed in post-mortems. This incidentally may explain the disagreeable stench given off by some chronic cases during the Fast. Putrefactive changes can also be noticed which explains the body odor. *The entire disease origin problem gravitates into the symptoms of blockage. Remove the obstruction and the channels and fibers of life throb into renewal activity and good health.*

The living organism must maintain its oxidizing mechanism in order to keep from dying. During the fast, the food now must come from within. The body economy now can accomplish chemical changes so perfectly as being unmatched by any other laboratory process. Uric acid can actually be transformed into protein, from whence it came. Cholesterol is reconverted to fat—carbonic acid changed to starch or sugar. It is the great transformation or operation without the knife which takes its course with the greatest of precision.

THE PROCESS OF AUTOLYSIS

The process of autolysis (self consumed) is inaugurated. All tissue components, not essential, are oxidized or burned in order to maintain life. This is the incredible manifestation of higher intelligence taking over command.

Many alterations can now be observed in the entrance to the digestive organs. Most noticeable is the coated tongue and disagreeable mouth odor. This unpleasant emanation does not come from the newly displayed phlegm but mostly from the lungs. Here we find body chemistry in a noble effort to bring about elimination of hardened infusion, liquified by the fast. This cleansing is carried out predominantly by the blood and lymph stream, using kidneys, bowels and skin as an exit for the dissolved wasted products.

The sometimes obnoxious odor could also come from partially degenerated organs undergoing dissolution. Last but not least the odor generally also originates in the colon, the great "sewer pipe" of the body. Sluggish bowel action, impacted fecal material could contribute by the production of noxious gases which in turn reach the lungs through osmosis to be removed to the outside through the breath. While fasting, it is advisable to stay away from people as much as possible. The coating from the tongue should be removed twice daily with a stiff toothbrush. The chewing of parsley or cinnamon bark will help to disguise the offensive breath.

ACTION OF THE STOMACH DURING THE FAST

Under a complete fast, where only water or herbal teas are consumed, hydrochloric acid production is greatly reduced. This is the one significant improvement to the juice diet in which stomach acidity is not always retarded. Consequently, hunger sensations may become prolonged, making the juice diet more difficult to withstand.

The first two or three days of the fast are the most trying to go through. After that, most hunger pangs disappear after which the individual seems to "float," strangely feeling free of many disagreeable sensations in the abdominal region. Buchinger reached this stage only after the fourth day when he stated that "everything became quiet on the Western front." Rumblings from fermentations lessens, all organs appear to greatly appreciate the new well deserved rest.

An important change in the stomach is its shrinkage during the fast. The normal healthy stomach in an adult is supposed to equal the size of two fists, holding a little more than one pint. That this is not the case in us "civilized" beings can be attested by all surgeons or morticians. I have seen stomachs in post-mortems measuring several times the normal size. Such distended stomachs have exceedingly thin walls resulting in defective function. In the prolonged fast, the shrinking process of the stomach goes on and stops, whenever the normal size has been regained.

THE GALL BLADDER

Here we may find drastic reactions to the sudden withdrawal of food. Secretions of gall continue to accumulate in this reservoir, in some cases in an increased tempo. The solution may often regurgitate into the stomach, giving rise to temporary spells of nausea or vomiting. The great Dr. Tilden used the stomach tube in such cases, emptying the stomach of its contents. The drinking of one pint of lukewarm water with insertion of finger into throat also answers the purpose, inducing emptying through vomiting.

THE PANCREAS

In the fast, the pancreas reduces in size. The functional integrity of the digestive portion of the gland is greatly enhanced. The endocrine part (Islands of Langerhans) often becomes so re-activated as to reduce implications of Diabetes.

The production of hormones or digestive ferments is somewhat sluggish immediately after the fast. It may take several days to bring about normal secretion, explaining the importance of breaking the fast.

THE SMALL AND LARGE INTESTINE

The small intestine also shrinks in both length and diameter. The colon, besides shrinking, undergoes a decided re-organization.

About 75% or three quarters in the amount of stool is made out of bacteria, dead or alive. It is interesting to learn that the colon may become completely sterile in a ten day fast. Still more significant is the problem of impacted feces. A British surgeon once made the statement that the average man carries with him such hardened bowel wastes to the extent of between several ounces to as much as *fifty pounds*. I have seen colons on the marble slab practically being rigidified with uneliminated retained stool. Only a small opening in the center permitted passage of some bowel content.

During the fast, the impactions clinging to the colon wall loosen, and copious stools are passed. This is one of the most perplexing experiences to a faster, when no food had been ingested.

HEART AND BLOOD VESSELS

The heart again assumes normal shape in the fast, vessels become freed of their clogging infusions (cholesterol). The average size of a well fed "civilized" heart is enlarged, which is now being corrected. The vessels and capillaries of the heart (coronary) receive a most thorough cleansing, restoring normal fluid circulation. It is also possible that the fast could absorb scar tissue formations in cases of rheumatic heart conditions. How else could one explain the amazing improvements achieved by the fast in such cases?

As to abnormal Blood pressure, it is amazing how quickly and efficiently the fast comes to the rescue. High pressure ratings lower from day to day—most likely due to the absorption of cholesterol. In the case of abnormal low pressure, the explanation is more difficult. Undoubtedly, the adrenal glands are involved, where functional integrity is brought about by the fast.

THE PULSE

The pulse is usually increased at the start, then falls below normal as the fast continues. Rates may vary from forty to one-hundred-twenty beats per minute, which may become erratic from time to time.

Should the pulse remain irregular for longer periods, or when extreme low or high pulse rate prevail, the fast should be broken.

THE BLOOD

While the quantity of the blood volume is reduced in proportion to loss of body weight, the quality of the blood is greatly improved during the fast. It is amazing to observe the gradual increase of red cells in the blood picture.

Dr. Weger and Dr. Tilden reported cases of pernicious anemia where the red count doubled in periods from one week to twelve days. The abnormal high white count had also been reduced two and one-half times during these observations.

The primary reason for anemia accordingly is not nutritional deficiency, but cellular obstruction in organs and glands preventing *utilization* of the food. The blood building mechanism in bone marrow, liver, spleen, etc. is put into a higher degree of perfection by the cleansing action of the fast. This does not mean that nutrition is of no consequence to the relative state of the blood. This, however, is always secondary—improper body chemistry coming first. This is why many top European sanatoriums inaugurate dietary reforms with temporary food withholding.

THE LUNGS

The gradual absorption of mucus from the miles of hair like tubes in the lungs make deep and effortless breathing a most pleasant experience to the faster. The voice becomes clear and resonant.

The fast does provide an excellent opportunity to practice deep breathing. In some of such experiments it was established that the volume of breath intake (air) doubled. In connection with skin brushing with dry brush great improvements in the general oxidizing mechanism of the body can be attained.

THE SKIN

The skin as well as the teeth are the parts that reveal a true indication of body condition.

With the lowering of metabolic efficiency, the skin becomes pale, thin and dry with development of many folds. Secretions of perspiration lessen with an increasing difficulty of keeping warm.

During the fast, the skin resumes more effectively its role of body cleanser. Perspiration may become odoriferous as it may carry dissolved particles of uric acid, decomposed cells, etc.

One of the most gratifying effects of the fast is the observance of changes of the skin. The once shiny cigarette paper appearance, particularly on extremities, change over to a more velvety texture, the skin loses its shine and many folds, and becomes thicker.

THE KIDNEYS AND BLADDER

Constituting the great filter apparatus of the body, it can be seen that the kidneys participate greatly in this new effort of body reorientation. At the start of the fast, the urine is invariably dark in color, strongly acid in reaction, and of high specific gravity. Dissolved uric acid, phosphates and bile pigment are making up the ingredients responsible for the relative "thickness" of the urine. The odor may become offensive.

As the fast progresses, the color of the urine becomes lighter, being less odoriferous. This improvement in urinary characteristics is in direct proportion to the amount of cellular waste being "melted" out of the body structures. It must be remembered that next to the colon, the kidneys carry the largest load in the removal of metabolic waste from the body.

To fully appreciate the benefits bestowed by a fast to the urinary system, one should follow a typical case. A male patient came to me, complaining of constant burning sensation in region of bladder, as well as having to get up every hour at night to urinate. The patient submitted to a twelve day fast, after which all burning sensations disappeared and the man slept through the entire night.

Buchinger made a thorough study of this kidney-bladder phenomenon and broadly speaks of specific anti-bodies produced by the body during the fast. Accordingly, the fasting organism in its concentration on worn out or diseased tissues, manufactures certain "medicinal" agents from the diseased organs to be used in the healing or repair of such organs. This protective mechanism partially explains seemingly impossible correction of long existing disease processes. Other investigators have corroborated Buchinger's assertions and claim the faster's urine to be virtually a healing concoction.

Incidentally, Buchinger's first patient, a woman physician, aborted a handful of kidney stones after an eleven day fast.

THE ENEMA AND THE FAST

Contrary to the opinion of some fasting authorities in the U.S., the temporary use of the enema during the fast is not only desirable, but highly essential. I have come to this conclusion after having studied the problem in a life time of work on thousands of patients. The European fasting experts with their traditional thoroughness for detail and scientific reasoning also have concluded that this "emergency" clearing procedure of the intestinal tract during the fast to be a most important provision for achieving best results.

From a purely functional point of view, the greatest amount of discarded waste is "dumped" into the colon. Since there is no bulk connected with this excretion, contractile movements of the "gut" can hardly be expected. The resulting "dormancy" in the intestine does permit some re-absorption of the highly toxic material into the blood stream, often explaining severe headaches experienced during the fast.

This is most convincingly demonstrated when such agonizing headaches miraculously disappear while taking the enema. A standard rubber enema bag holding two quarts most amply fulfills the purpose. Best position is knee-chest. Bag is tied with string to door knob, medicine chest or wherever string can be applied. Regulate distance between bag and "inlet" to about two and one-half feet. In knee-chest position breathe (pant) deeply, thus affording intestinal relaxation. Water temperature is slightly below that of body (96°). Control flow of water by pinching tube with fingers. If too much distress is experienced during inflow of water, squeeze off tube but maintain heavy breathing. Soon discomfort will leave, to permit more water to flow into colon.

Try to hold as much water as possible and gently massage abdomen before emptying at the toilet. This procedure may have to be repeated once or more times for a more intensive internal cleansing.

Molasses or honey may be included to achieve greater osmotic attraction (two tablespoons per quart). Also flaxseed teas and sea-water have been used in cases of inflammatory processes in the colon.

ACID—ALKALINE BALANCE

Since the fasting organism is literally feeding on its own substance, that is, fat and protein, it is logically assumed that a decided acid reaction or acidosis would be the result. This is entirely erroneous, as anyone experienced with fasting can testify.

The famous Dr. Haig expressed it succinctly: "fasting acts like a dose of alkali."

During the fast the body lives on its reserves. Alkaline reacting minerals are liberated and shifted to other parts of the body. Calcium and potassium are retained longer than sulphur or phosphorous to maintain chemical balance. This does not mean that in some isolated cases during short spells a slight case of acidosis may develop. This could be considered a crisis and rarely lasts more than a day or two.

BODY CHANGES CAUSED BY AUTOLYSIS

In the fast, autolysis accounts for the remarkable changes taking place in the body. It was Dr. Sylvester Graham who wrote over a century ago that "it is a general law of autolysis to first remove those substances which are of least use to the economy; and hence, all morbid accumulations, such as wens, tumors, abscesses during the fast."

Dr. Trall remarked that abnormal growths possess a lower grade of vitality than normal growths, thus are easiest to destroy. In my own experience I have seen many times lumps under skin (fatty tumors) as well as in breasts shrink and often completely disappear. With mathematical precision one can expect a tumorous mass to shrink during the fast. However, some types of abnormal growths do not always entirely disappear, such as fibroids in the female. There exist other and deeper implications of the disorder brought about by disorganized sex practice, emotional instabilities, etc.

LENGTH OF THE FAST

There are two schools of thought about the length of the fast. Some advocate short fasts of up to seven days, others claim that only nature should indicate when to resume eating. This indication is the return of hunger, cleansing of tongue and breath, etc.

There is no question that the prolonged fast is the most effective and—strange as it seems—the easiest to undergo. If healing crises do occur, they usually are of short duration. The rest of time the body is seemingly "floating" in space. The time elements of such "long" fasts range from ten to as long as thirty days. The European fasting institutes try to limit the fast to twenty-one days and only reluctantly agree to go for longer periods.

In this connection, a word of caution should be in place. A prolonged fast should always be conducted under the supervision of a physician trained in this therapy in suitable surroundings.

This does not mean that the short fast of five to six days is of no benefit to the health seeker. Such short food withholdings can be carried out at home, often without interruption to established work schedule, particularly by those of robust constitution. In cases of well developed chronic disorders, these fasts can be repeated every three or four weeks for from three to five or more times.

Assuming that a chronic disorder requires thirty days of fasting, dividing it into several stages of five days, would require six—five day fasts. This sort of calculation, however, is not quite correct as a certain amount of momentum is lost by the various interruptions. One decided advantage to the "stage" faster can be observed: A remarkable improvement of character trends and habit pattern. There is no question that the voluntary submission to a fast requires a great amount of will power or mental fortitude.

The renewed self disciplinary actions open up hidden reservoirs of mental and spiritual potentials in the faster, which now in a mysterious way reveal deeper significances to living. Slowly, but inexorably, the *faster becomes a philosopher.*

SAFETY OF THE FAST

The majority of European fasting experts are well trained medical doctors who became attracted to the healing force of the fast by observing speedy corrections of diseased conditions in others or in themselves. About the safety features of the fast, all authorities agree that it is the safest healing method known. One case in Germany attracted some publicity—a patient deliberately committed suicide by taking prolonged over-heated baths during the fast.

Otherwise, there have been practically no fatalities in several hundred thousand cases, an enviable record. This becomes more apparent when considering the severity of conditions of those patients who often cling to the fast in a last effort for help.

Of course it is possible that a sick person may die while fasting. Because of the prevailing ignorance about the subject, some sick person may not turn to fasting until becoming desperate. Possibly the degeneration of vital organs had been too far advanced.

Otherwise, death from fasting is not possible until the body has lost at least one-third of its normal weight. In an average case this would require sixty days or more of fasting—more accurately now termed starving.

Even so, there are cases of obesity on record, where fasting periods have been extended to as long as one-hundred and fifty days without apparent damage to the faster. At any rate, the European record speaks for itself—with safety features unparalleled by any other healing method.

NEGATIVE INDICATORS FOR FASTING

1. Extremely emaciated patients should not fast longer than up to three days at a time, with intervals of constructive diets.

These short fasts can be repeated until the emaciation is overcome.

2. Advanced cases of tuberculosis or malignancies.

Some U. S. experts advise against fasting in advanced osteoarthritis with bone degeneration, advanced diabetes, general wasting disease and lead poisoning. In Europe, contra-indications to the fact are held to a minimum.

GENERAL SUGGESTIONS FOR STARTING THE FAST

It is advisable to prepare for the fast by first changing the diet to exclusive fruit diet two or three days before the beginning of the fast. Tarty apples seem to answer best the purpose —about two pounds per day. The ingested apples act as a broom in the digestive tube. A laxative is taken in the evening of the last fruit day to be followed with daily enemas during the first days of the fast.

Factors to Watch On Starting a Fast

There are many reasons why some individuals do not take advantage from the great benefits that can be expected from an occasional abstention of food.

Fear of the fast is the greatest handicap one must overcome, that is why it is so essential to study or read about the fast as much as possible.

Next, we find it extremely difficult to go even *without* a single meal, what I prefer to call the "euphoria addiction." Furthermore, there are many of us who find it abhorrent to deviate from the accepted "Jones pattern" of living. What would my friends or relatives say "if I would starve myself" is often given as an important reason to maintain the "status quo."

The following suggestions have proven to overcome the various objections to the fast. Let us start by withholding food only for a single day. It was Goethe who said "that anything *immediately started is already half done.*" Water only or herbal teas would be preferable, but for some of us who are more apprehensive, juices from grape, apple or orange, up to three pints, could be taken. At the end of the first day, let us closely scrutinize our appearance and feeling. Let us look into a mirror and examine our tongue. Does it appear pink and smooth, or does it look grey, heavily coated with mucus? What is the odor of the breath, is it wholesome or tainted? How about the eyes, are they clear or do they seem to have "spots" floating in them? Many of such drastic changes in appearance and functions of body can be noted after but a single day of fasting, even on the fruit regimen.

It is obvious that such demonstrable changes experienced by ourselves in the span of but twenty-four hours is utterly convincing. Our reasoning faculties become aroused. All of us are aware that where there is smoke, there must be fire.

With great fascination we note the immediate mobilization of body command. The display of waste removal and odoriferousness of breath leaves no doubt in our mind about the thoroughness of reorganization, controlled by an unerring intelligence.

The first day without food has passed, surprisingly we do not feel too bad—but in any case have made a great discovery —that there is more to our existence than "by bread alone." The first day of this new experience has removed great doubts and fears about the fast and has sparked a flaming desire to learn more about the intrinsic potentials of our being. Many of us wish to continue another or more days on the fast, as we instinctively feel the great need and blessing of this amazing inner corrective force, generated by the fast.

AN INCREDIBLE EXPERIENCE IN ENFORCED FASTING

In March 1963, all World news media highlighted the experience of a forty-two year old man and a twenty-one year old co-ed in the wilderness of Northern Canada. Following a plane smash-up, the couple had been rescued after having been isolated during the coldest season for forty-nine days, subsiding on a few emergency food rations for a few days and over one entire month with no food at all.

The weight losses were forty pounds for the man and thirty pounds for the young lady. To help the monotony of the diet of water, the co-ed remarked, "we drank it three ways: hot, cold and boiled."

After the rescue, the couple was examined by physicians who found them to be in "remarkably good condition."

A FASTING MARCH IN SWEDEN

Eleven members of the Swedish Vegetarian Society and Waerland movement started a fast march on August 1, 1954 from Goeteburg to Stockholm. It was attempted to make the trip of 325 miles in ten days without taking any food whatsoever, walking an average of 32.5 miles per day on a complete fast except the drinking of spring water.

Ten of the eleven members reached Stockholm according to schedule, in perfect physical condition, with elastic steps.

The purpose of the group March was a mass demonstration of the relative safety of the fast, even when undertaken during periods of extreme body exertions. The demonstration became a huge success. Hundreds of thousands of people lined the streets of towns passed by the marchers. Several physicians participated "part time" in the march who kept a close control of the fasters during the trip. Most of the days it rained heavily without let-up. In spite of it, the goal and objective was reached in the allotted time. The members marched in training clothes and sandals. The average weight loss was a little less than two pounds per day.

The physicians in the largest hospital in Stockholm immediately examined all fasters and were astounded about the excellent health status of each member.

The Swedish press at the start was somewhat reserved, if not hostile about the undertaking. But in a matter of a few days a decided change was noted in all of the Swedish papers. The new orientation was that of complete understanding in this "drastic display of mobilizing forces not as yet recognized to improve the general health status of an entire nation."

One paper remarked that the reception of the fasters was

"fantastic, a triumph with three times the number of people lining the streets as in royal receptions."

Dr. Ragner Berg, the great Nutrition expert and Nobel Prize Winner wrote that he was not surprised about the good results achieved by the demonstration. He also stated that he knew of fasts of over one hundred days duration and that we need not fear of dying from hunger. He also mentioned having supervised or controlled fasts up to six weeks. He himself fasted often up to twenty-one days, working eleven hours daily in laboratory or at desk. However, he felt that the march was a great scientific success in that it created a true valuation of the fast in millions of people.

THE BREAKING OF THE FAST

In short fasts up to six days, we need not become too much concerned about the breaking of the fast. More important is the type of food, amount and manner of eating. Foods should be shunned that are of animal origin, foods high of concentration or food subjected to refinement or synthetics.

All fasting experiences always create a new alertness or apprehension for quality instigated by the improved organism. The protective mechanism of instinct is re-awakened or strengthened in direct proportion to the amount of cleansing action (duration) of the fast. A gradual but irresistible change in taste sensations becomes apparent—new cravings develop toward the simple and natural foods, fruits, nuts, (seeds) and vegetables. Strikingly paralleled with this new eating orientation is the new discovery that raw, uncooked members of this category are not only more nutritious, but equally better tasting.

Our first food day consequently should start with fruit or vegetable juice, two or three pints per day. I prefer grape juice but the juices from orange, grapefruit, apple or pear could be substituted. On second day start with juice, or whole fruit for breakfast. Noon and evening always include large portions of raw vegetable salads. Gradually try to adhere to eating pattern as suggested in dietary chapter.

The breaking of longer fasts is more important. As a general rule, each five days of complete food abstinence require one day of fruit or vegetable juice. The hormone glands of entire digestive apparatus are not functioning or only partially so at the start of ingestion. Several days may be required for the reactivation of all components needed for food assimilation.

The chewing of the food now becomes urgent of consideration. Dr. Fletcher many years ago proved that thorough mastication (fletcherizing) of food could decidedly improve general body conditions even without regard to the type of quality of the food. Each bite of food morsel should be chewed thirty to forty times until completely liquified. It is asserted that with less food better assimilation is achieved with a remarkable absence of abdominal discomfort (lack of gas forming tendencies). Let us try this new chewing "ritual" for a few days and prove to ourselves the trueness of Dr. Fletcher's discovery.

FRUIT JUICE DIETS

There appear to be some misconceptions about the meaning of water fast, juice fasts and so forth. Literally, water fast means abstinence from water, juice fast-abstinence of juice, vegetable fast-abstinence from vegetables, etc., etc.

What is applied to fasting in these pages relates to abstinence to food, except water. Various types of herbal teas could be taken in place of water. In this case we have water plus some aromatic substances as found in some herbs such as mint, orange blossom, alfalfa, linden blossom, sage, etc. The addition of these herbal agents does not necessarily change the effectiveness of the "water only" restrictions. It does, however, improve the otherwise flat taste of the water. Also, during the cold season, the fluid can be taken in a heated condition, which is more palatable than plain water. In cases of temporary weakness, the patient can add some honey to the tea, making the drink more delightful.

As to the "juice fast": What is obviously meant is abstention from food except fruit or vegetable juices. Such a juice diet could be of great help if carried out over a few days several times each month. To go longer than three or four days on a juice diet is not advised because of two reasons:

1. Since juices are partial foods, certain secretions in the stomach continue to be manufactured such as hydrochloric acid. In the absence of solid foods (proteins), the acid often begins to digest the stomach wall itself, creating ulcers.

2. Because of the continuity of digestive secretions (even partial) hunger sensations are apt to be prolonged. In my many years of fasting experience I have repeatedly observed the superiority of the water diet to that of the juice. In the former, there are few, if any complications, in less than three days all food cravings disappear, making the faster feel strangely free of all "earthbound" attachments.

Yet, the fruit diet could be of help in cases of extreme emaciation or where it is difficult to go more than a few days without food.

The juices of grape, orange, grapefruit, or apple have proven to give best results. Amounts of between two to three pints per day are recommended. Water in addition can be taken, as desired.

SPECIFIC ENEMA TECHNIQUES

The enema became focused into national prominence when a successful U. S. baby specialist became embroiled in a professional dispute.

The enema, using epsom salt water, was the controversial treatment for a disease that kills 25,000 infants in the U. S. each year. The malady is called *hyaline membrane disease*. It was this disorder which killed the infant son of the late President Kennedy, in 1963.

The doctor who "discovered" the epsom salt enema treatment claimed that this bowel cleansing method had saved 28 babies. He described the effects of the treatment as most dramatic. Babies that were suffocating became "normal" in an hour or less.

"It's a silly thing to use epsom salt enemas in this age of modern medicine" the doctor declared. "It's a silly thing, but it works. I know it seems ridiculous and I can still hardly believe it myself. But many people by now have seen that it works."

So spoke the doctor who became amazed about a basic procedure known, practiced and suggested by every drugless or Naturopathic doctor throughout the world.

Colon hygiene combats the beginning of decay, propagation of disease germs and the spreading of toxin at the very source. In the case of the suffocating babies, the self generated poisons had been washed out of the colon before they could spread and paralyze the nerves of respiration (diaphragm).

By the use of the enema, the doctor had saved the lives of 28 babies. But the eminent hospital staff was unimpressed. They called the enema treatment too "controversial" to be used. As an aftermath, the doctor quit his position at the hospital with the interpretation of the situation that he was fired.

In this connection, a few observations about the enema are in place. Essentially, the procedure is a cleansing process of the large intestine so highly rewarding to the user. Contrary to the opinion of some hygienists, the enema is not injurious and is not habit forming. There is no other means available for man to afford such speedy relief from headaches or other aches and pains created by metabolic disturbances than the occasional cleansing of the colon. Anyone can make the experiment and will immediately become convinced that the majority of headaches diminish in severity or completely disappear with the use of the enema. I may even go farther maintaining that in case of headaches, pain sensation will begin to abate *not only after but even during* the taking of the enema. That is how effective this internal hygiene measure operates.

The consensus of medical experts in Europe practicing the Naturopathic method in the healing approach is unanimous as to according hygienic attention to the intestinal tract. It would be unthinkable for them to supervise a fast of their patients without stressing the importance of the enema. With characteristic scientific thoroughness, these experts have amassed incontestable evidence that functional apparitions in the colon are behind nearly every constitutional disease.

There is a World famous European clinic, where practically

every disease under the sun in being treated primarily with detoxification of the digestive tube.

In my own experience, I have seen patients who presented sorry pictures of advanced body deterioration. In some cases, a few of these patients had been subjected to lengthy fasts without concern to the disposition of the colon. Quite often, an amazing improvement in both appearance and feeling of the patient had been achieved with the removal of toxic waste products that had been lodged or permitted to accumulate in pockets or convolutions in this big sewer-like organ of waste removal, the colon.

As previously discussed, the usual enema container holds two quarts. It is advisable to use sea water if obtainable or regular tap water to which is added two tablespoons of either molasses, honey, brown sugar or epsom salt. Also tea made out of flaxseed, one-half cup boiled in two quarts of water for twenty minutes, could be used in case of extreme mucous membrane involvements (colitis).

The knee-chest position is most adaptable. Container is fastened two and one-half feet above inlet. A string can be used to adjust the exact height from an object such as a door frame, etc. Nozzle of tube is slightly lubricated with K-Y jelly (water soluble), obtainable in drug stores. The tube is pinched with fingers of one hand to control amount of flow. While panting or breathing deeply through mouth, fluid is permitted to enter colon without creating too much discomfort. As soon as amount appears to be excessive, retract nozzle and empty colon content in stool.

An extremely important adjunct at this point should be suggested. There are many pockets, convolutions or tight areas of the colon demonstrable in many individuals. It is obvious that these abnormal colon conditions constitute hindrances to effective cleansing. A specific manipulation will help to overcome this. With water still in the abdomen raise both legs on chair, bed or against wall while lying on the back. With both hands firmly massage entire abdominal region, permitting the flow of liquid to reach obstructed areas as well as helping to disengage hardened fecal accumulations.

At the start the two quart enema may not be tolerated, in which case it may have to be taken in stages.

It will be found that repeated enema procedures will drastically improve painful and irritating sensations as evidenced by its curative effect.

During the fast, the enema may be taken once every day. Gradually it can be reduced to be taken every other day, then twice a week until no longer required.

It must be remembered, however, that the maintenance of abundant health requires constant vigilance. In obtaining this objective, the enema "ritual" will be found to be of great help.

Chart No. 7 is a schematic drawing of the digestive tract. In taking the enema, it will be helpful to study the drawing and become familiar with the structure of this ingenious mechanism of assimilation.

In Sec. 12 we find the rectum which is the end of the colon. But for our purpose it is the beginning of the irrigating process to be commenced. It is attempted to reach all around the horseshoe-like convoluted tube, up, around and down to the cecum indicated by Sec. 6.

Below Sec. 6 you find Sec. 5 outlining the appendix. This most strategic position is often the site of infection as here we find the most concentrated array of bacterial proliferation. In an inelegant term it could be called the cesspool of the body.

The Sec. 7 position is of importance since here we find the ileocecal valve. This consists of two flaps of tissue extending from the small intestine into the colon and intended by nature to permit but a one-way passage, from the small intestine, to the colon.

Sec. 11 represents the sum total of the small intestines in which food assimilation is accorded by fermentation.

Returning to Sec. 7 location we can see the importance of this little valve preventing the traveling of bacteria outside the assigned habitat, the colon.

The purpose of this diagram is to convey to us the serious implications that are associated with auto-intoxication. Because of abnormalities affecting the cecum such as bloating, distention, etc., the ileocecal valve remains open, permitting putrefactive bacteria invading the small intestines and from there reach organs such as duodenum, Sec. 4, gall bladder, Sec. 3, pancreas, Sec. 13, etc.

Post-mortem examinations have revealed the findings of these disease causing bacteria in all of these organs mentioned. In addition, the germs have been found in practically every every other organ including liver, heart and vessels.

It is the dramatic experience of the enterprising doctor, who used the enema and saved 28 babies out of the 25,000 cases that die every year. Remember his astonishment when he reported that within a period of one hour after the enema, the miracle took place, the suffocating babies could again breathe normally.

In the case of hyaline membrane disease described above, the effects of the germs or their toxic excretion resulted in suffocation of the babies by reaching up to the diaphragm and nerve supply of the lungs.

The "silly thing" of the enema promptly arrested the potential killers *at their breeding* ground before they could depart to their field of action.

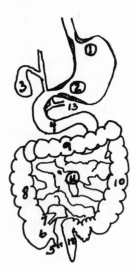

1. Cardiac Stomach
2. Pylorus
3. Gall bladder
4. Duodenum
5. Appendix
6. Cecum
7. Ileo-cecal valve
8. Ascending Colon
9. Transverse Colon
10. Descending (Sigmoid) Colon
11. Small Intestines
12. Rectum
13. Pancreas

Digestive Tract. Chart No. 6

4

Food —
Its Relations to Aches and Pains

Historical Nutritional Milestones

Many years ago, Commodore Perry had convinced the Japanese to open their ports to the Western powers. With unforeseen display of energies, the Japanese not only paralleled the organizational talent of the Western conquerors, but actually surpassed them.

In less than two decades, a once insignificant appearing small nation built a modern Army and Navy. So powerful became this aggressive force, that fifty years later the oriental midget succeeded in preventing the Russian colossus from grasping a portion of the East. In May 1905, Russia's once proud fleet burned and sank in the Korea Straits.

The old Czarist Empire was on the way out, and a new great power was born.

All of this is known to the World except the name of Takati. Without Takati, there would not have been the unbelievable construction of the Japanese Navy enabling it to destroy the giant Russian intruder. Yet Takati was neither admiral, general or politician, he was an insignificant physician attached to the Japanese Navy.

When Japan began to emulate Western concepts of military might, industry and commerce as introduced by Perry, it was inevitable that the "blessings" of food refinement was included. When twenty years later Japan did astound the World with its formidable Navy and Army copied from the conquerors, these amazing developments to a major power practically came to a standstill. A strange, crippling epidemic struck down the crew of the ships. A great number of the stricken men died, those who recovered, were unfit for further service.

Pasteur had just published his work on microbes (1878) which was eagerly accepted in Japan, where epidemics were suffered with regularity for centuries. Now, the specific bacillus had to be found. Symptoms were all the same. First great debility—nervous disorders, heart weakness, swelling of liver, loss of weight, paralysis and—death. The disease, Beriberi, became well known to Takati who often had three fourths of the crew in sick bay, with a mortality of forty percent.

Since the search for the causative bacillus was unsuccessful, Takati began to think about other possible causes. What about the food the men were eating? Could there be a connection with the strange malady?

His superiors wanted no part of this orientation—their stern order—"keep on looking for the bacillus" and continue to treat the sick and leave the feeding of our men to the commissary department. But the progress of the epidemic kept on. With clocklike precision the crews became sick, the ships helplessly anchored—the exciting advance movement of the Japanese Navy came to an abrupt stop.

But Takati was persistent. Finally, in despair, the Navy command gave in. Two naval vessels, each with three hundred men aboard, were ordered on a long cruise. One of the ships received the customary ration of polished rice. The other ship was supplied with rations used on British ships—that is oatmeal, vegetables, fish, meat and condensed milk.

As can be surmised, the rice diet ship resembled a hospital ship. More than two-thirds of the crew had come down with beriberi; on the other ship, the sailors were in good condition. Only four of the men had succumbed to the disease. When interrogated, they frankly admitted of having secretly partaken of the rice.

The Japanese Navy promptly reacted to the findings of the patient little doctor. In the rice supply, only the natural variety with its outer layer intact, was permitted to act as food.

It is significant for us to remember the date of this decision. The calendar shows that about 1880, man learned this important nutritional secret from Nature. The International Press duly disseminated this alarming information to all parts of the World. With strange apathy the frightening implications of the message was ignored. More epidemics had to follow—millions more had to suffer before learning by a painful search the price one must pay for food refinement.

You may ask what about now? The answer is obvious. From all appearances man does not always make use of his logical deductions. Polished rice is still sold by our processors—for that matter even served as partial food for the sick.

THE CHICKEN EXPERIMENT OF SUMATRA

The year was 1883, three years after the Japanese discovery. The Dutch Army doctor Christian Eijkman was ordered to go to the torrid jungle of Dutch East India to investigate beriberi, the mystifying problem of the colonial administrators. While the insurgent natives were unscathed by the disease, it was rampant in those regions under the control of the Dutch. This was contrary to the doctrine of Science that the epidemic should be more prevalent in regions where better hygiene prevailed.

Eijkman found that chickens fed with polished rice fell ill with beriberi—but could be cured with natural rice. It is said that the doctor wore out a flock of chickens by making them repeatedly sick and well again.

WELL MEANING LADIES BRING BERIBERI
TO THE PHILIPPINES

The year is 1898. The United States won the war with Spain and found herself in possession of the Philippines.

The American administrators, missionaries and doctors brought their wives with them. This female contingent found many opportunities for social work on the island. There were many things that appeared in need of improvement to these nice ladies with their delicate white complexions.

In particular they were shocked by the natural rice of the natives, unequal in size, dirty looking as to color, with large unappetizing kernels. Immediately, the wheels of civilized food reform were put into high gear.

The "lowly" primitive rice grain received first attention. Modern refining machinery was introduced. The ugly kernel was freed from its husk and polished a number of times during which process the silvery protective skin and the seed sprout were removed. After further polishings, the kernels were glazed with talcum, they were now equal in size, white as snow, smooth as china.

The good ladies could relax now, a part of their objectives had been attained. The ugly ducklings had been transformed into graceful swans. Polite society no longer had to blush in embarrassment when confronted with the staple diet of the natives.

Then slowly, but unrelentingly the effects of the food reform appeared. People became sick in proportion to their intake of the refined rice. Beriberi assumed epidemic proportions.

It was not until 1902 when Takati's report was taken seriously. The prison fare of polished rice was changed again to the despised natural rice. In due time, Beriberi was eradicated.

THE LESSONS LEARNED BY SAILORS

Ancient seafarers not only had to battle the elements of the sea and winds, a far greater danger was imbedded in contracting *Scurvy*. This disease started with bleeding of the gums and inflammation of the jaw. The teeth became loose and fell out. At a later stage internal hemorrhages began with dropsical swelling of the legs.

Vasco da Gama, while sailing around the Cape of Good Hope in 1498, lost two-thirds of his crew and nearly failed to complete the trip.

It was found that all signs of the disease would quickly vanish with the intake of lemons and oranges. For this reason, the British Navy, under Admiral Hawkins in the 16th Century, made citric fruits or their juices required nutritional supplement. It is interesting to note in this connection that the dreaded scurvy was not always prevented on long journeys with this juice protection.

In most cases, the juice therapy worked perfectly, in a few other cases it completely failed. This inconsistent, "Now it works, now it doesn't" discrepancy of expected results baffled the naval authorities for a long time, until the puzzle was solved. Some over-ambitious cooks wanted to improve the juice by boiling it. With unfailing precision, the citric juice promptly lost its healing or preventive properties with the appearance of scurvy.

Some old seafaring captains also noted that scurvy could be prevented in his crew or passengers, when freshly brewed beer was plentifully served. It was learned that the barley in the *sprouting process* develops certain organic matter which is effective to prevent scurvy. The Chinese have used this principle for many centuries by supplementing their meager diets with freshly *sprouted grains,* consumed without cooking. The story goes that this food habit was accidentally discovered over 2000 years ago. During a river journey a food scarcity evolved, there was nothing left but a sack of soy beans, thoroughly soaked. Since there was no other food left, it was decided to eat the "spoiled" beans, which were in a process of sprouting. The half starved people were surprised about the good taste of the sprouts. They aleso felt well nourished with this singular diet.

Today it is known that the content of protein in grains or legumes during sprouting is improved in the development of rare animo-acids, as well as general quality. Also, Vitamin A and C among other nutritional components, are generated. The sprouts are easy to digest, and are of an agreeable sweet taste.

This explains the amazing healing effect of this "5 day vegetable" in Nutritional deficiencies.

The use of sprouts of seeds, grains or legumes offers the most effective means of withstanding temporary stays in unhospitable climates (Arctic, desert, stony islands, high mountains). The "fresh food" requirement can thus be solved in a simple manner.

Another fascinating contribution in the food drama was made in 1734. In an English brig on the voyage to Greenland one of the sailors became so sick that it was assumed he could not survive. To prevent the spread of the disease, it was decided to get rid of the sailor. A small island was approached and the patient put ashore. In spite of his weakness and swollen legs, the poor wretch, driven by hunger, began to fill his mouth with fresh young grass found sprouting in various places.

The miracle took place. The candidate for oblivion cheated death—in a matter of a few days the man felt the return of strength. Soon he could sit up—then he found that he could walk again. By hunting for shell fish and snails, the doomed man now could balance his grass diet. A short time afterwards, he was picked up by a passing ship and returned to England.

The recovery of the "incurable" sailor was hailed as a true miracle. It is significant for us to note that this healing force imbedded in fresh plants was demonstrated over two-hundred and thirty years ago. How much longer must ignorance prevail to prolong the miseries of humanity?

It was the great inventor Kettering (automobile self starter, etc.) who so pointedly remarked: "It is the great tragedy of society that of its Scientists only one in a thousand has enough imagination to look beyond the blinkers, imposed by conformity."

Along this thought it is not surprising that much of this incontestable evidence pointing to nutritional deficiencies was ignored. How could it be explained otherwise when a most modernly and "scientifically" trained human group could fall into the same trap of food ignorance?

On April 11, 1915, the German cruiser "Kronprinz Wilhelm," after having successfully raided the seas for nearly thee quarters of a year, had to admit defeat by a far greater opponent— incapacitating disease and death.

A large number of the ship's crew had fallen prostrate on the deck—the others were on the verge of collapse. The ship anchored at Newport News, U.S.A., hoping to find a miraculous cure to save the men.

It was Alfred W. McCann, reporter of a New York paper and former health commissioner, who immediately diagnosed the epidemic as Scurvy. It is to the credit of Dr. Perrenon, the ship's chief surgeon, that McCann's precise recommendations were explicitly followed.

As a result, within ten days a large portion of affected men were cured, the others following quickly in completely overcoming the malady.

The treatment then had worked wonders. Of what, then, did it consist?

The sinking of so many French and British ships, yielded enormous quantities of meat, white flour, sugar, margarine, cheese, condensed milk, canned vegetables, ham, bacon, beer, wine and spirits. It was obvious to McCann as it should have been to anyone with common sense and a little knowledge of dietetics, that such a diet is badly deficient in Vitamins, Minerals, Enzymes, etc. Another important life substance was also missing, that of Auxone, needed for cell regeneration.

The canned vegetables in a fresh state would have been sufficient to prevent the disease, their life substances either were boiled away or had been lost through canning.

According to McCann, the lifeless food disorganized body chemistry. Specifically, it abstracted the lime salts from the fibrous tissues, muscles, nerves, cartilages and bones. The resulting swelling of the limbs was due to the increased vascularity, causing weakness, neuralgic pains and effusion into the joints.

McCann's device was to restore life elements, or those food components which had been removed by the refining process.

One hundred pounds of wheat bran were soaked in two hundred pounds of water for twelve hours at 120° F. Of this liquid every man was given eight ounces each morning. Of the bran itself, each man received one heaping teaspoon morning and night until the stool became loose. A soup was made from spinach, onions, turnips, cabbage and carrots, only the liquid part consumed with dry whole wheat bread.

Potatoes were washed and peeled—their skins retained and boiled, the rest discarded. Again, the liquid part was used and given as a drink, four ounces to each man a day.

In addition, each man received the yolk of an egg every three hours in fresh, sweet milk.

In between time, the juice of ripe oranges was served. Apples were kept available to the men at all times.

As can be seen, the corrective diet excluded all the highly touted niceties of "foodless" foods, so eagerly hoarded by the ships' commissary and—so generously displayed in our markets not only then, but even now.

There lies the deep tragedy, modern man simply refuses to learn the lessons from past mistakes.

It was in the Sixteenth Century, when Sir William Gilbert said, "Science has done its utmost to prevent whatever Science has done."

In the field of Nutrition, so much has been learned about the part it is playing in providing optimum well-being for man or beast. Papers and books have been written by the tons to put down all the findings of this painstaking search. And yet, ninety percent of all people are sick as corroborated many times by similar painstaking researchers. A large portion of this sick segment in Westernized countries suffer from borderline degrees of beriberi, scurvy and other deficiency diseases.

One of our best beloved actors died of malnutrition (stomach ailment) in this the richest country of the globe. Radio and television constantly blare the blessings of pills and portions for "tired blood," or "bad nerves." With nauseating repetition we are reminded about the benefits of concoctions that make us able to endure "those aches and pains."

Admittedly something must be wrong with our food pattern. The commercial octopus has firmly entrenched itself with this frightening process of changing health provoking natural foods to the prevailing phony counterparts.

While traveling, this sorry nutrition picture becomes increasingly difficult to withstand. Excepting buttermilk and raw salads, very little can be obtained in the line of natural nutrients. Trains and airlines serve well-prepared dishes, catering to the tastes and demands of people, ninety percent of whom are sick, undoubtedly made so by the food.

It is extremely difficult to deviate from the dictum, "when in Rome, do as the Romans do" since there is hardly any opportunity to sidestep this behavior pattern. In food, the emphasis is richness, particularly animal protein, coffee and highballs.

Things are a little better in Canada. Delicious bran muffins are obtainable in most restaurants. South of the Rio Grande, delectable fruits and many natural corn meal varieties are plentiful for the traveler in countless places—all the way down into South America.

The situation in Europe is speedily improving. The better eating establishments offer both conventional and "reform" fare. In the latter and more expensive variety, the production of the food is tended along recent findings, starting from the very beginning of production—the soil. Terms such as "Freedom from chemical fertilizer or poisonous sprays" are incorporated as part of the menu. Vegetable or fruit juices prepared by a special process without disturbance of nutritional qualities, are offered. Vegetarian dishes, with unfired fruit and vegetables have become stylish. Whole grain bread or rolls in all varieties are available.

In Finland and Russia, the food picture is possibly the healthiest outside small regions in Asia and Africa. Unpasteurized milk from healthy cows can be obtained most everywhere in Finland. Traveling through that lovely country is a delight, particularly so, when one considers the enjoyment of the Sauna bath, with which no Finnish town or community would be without.

In Russia, the good, sturdy rye bread is made from grain fully ripened in the field. Then there is the national dish borsch, made from beets and cabbage, often in a partially fermented (sour) state.

This is possibly the reason for grave concern among European nutrition experts about the respective future of Eastern and Western cultures. There exists an enviable vitality and vigor among the masses of our Eastern neighbors. Continuing on our Eastern trek we may pass through the Caucasian or European segment of the East and slip into the Oriental portion or Far East.

Here we may find the real cause of apprehension, when pondering about the awakening of a sleeping colossus which in foreseeable times will number nearly one billion people. This cautious impression becomes more valid when considering racial character trends of stoicism and survival talents to hostilities, shortly in grasp of the hydrogen bomb.

I am referring to the Chinese, who, through thousands of years, have maintained a relatively high physical strength. This general freedom from disease is the more surprising in view of their dominant vegetarian diet. The daily meat ration of fifteen grams against the American one-hundred-twenty grams of course is only of statistical significance. A small segment of the Chinese population eats more than the average portion, while the Chinese peasant is practically a vegetarian.

Besides not having too much meat, the Chinese peasant lacks another source of protein, that of milk. But a vegetarian milk, obtained from soybeans is so becoming, that even children can digest it. The strict adherence to sprouting of grains and legumes also helps to supplement this meager fare.

When traveling through China, before the takeover by the Communists, I was often amazed by the excellent health status of the rural population. In the large cities, however, the impact of modern concepts of industrialization and food processing inevitably would respond in a decidedly reduced display of vitality in their people. Polished rice and refined grains, the latter frequently coming from the U.S. was often the cause of their plight. If it hadn't been for small amounts of vegetables and soy products, occasional flare-ups of beri-beri epidemics would have resulted.

THE WAERLAND MOVEMENT

In our study of following the history of human development, we became acquainted with the lives of some important personalities, who were able to influence the course of events. Going back many years, we find Hippocrates, known as the father of medicine. It is quite possible that this outstanding doctor became greatly influenced by another great man, Pythagoras, who died in 500 B.C., forty years before the birth of Hippocrates (460 B.C.).

Philosophies based on ethics, moral concepts and vegetarianism were the teachings of Pythagoras, so intensely emulated by Hippocrates.

Slowly the centuries went by. The human mind sank into the quagmire of supersitition and religious dogma. Book burnings brought on the long intellectual sleep of the middle age. Modern times erupted in two World Wars, racial and national barriers began to shrink. The march of disease and degeneration took bigger strides. Inquisitive minds started to ask pertinent questions about causes and how to get well. In some vulgar terms it was said that at the age of forty, man is either an idiot or his own physician.

The cry of the masses for a new healing concept brought on the medical revolution in Central Europe in treatment orientations as exemplified by Buchinger, Bircher-Benner, Kollath, etc.

While most medical reformers adopted the new treatment and nutrition approach through need to heal their own diseased bodies—the acceptance to the masses had already been prepared. There were two powerful personalities, responsible for the acceptance of this new thought about nutrition. One started out as a student, the other as a full-fledged physician. Both men were desperately sick and searching for health. One of the men came from Sweden, the other from Switzerland. Waerland was the one from the North, developing into a master orator able to condition the mass mind with his convincing logic.

A few years ago, Waerland passed away (due to an accident) at the age of eighty. But the memory of this great man will live on as long as humanity prevails.

In my estimation, Waerland has accomplished more than MacFadden in the U.S. in bringing a true health message to many thousands. His painstaking research and clear deductions could no longer be ignored by the masses or by scientifically trained minds.

At this time, there are countless followers and a great number of Waerland institutes, where serious or so-called incurable disease conditions are successfully overcome. The chief treatment is fasting and strict adherence to a specific diet.

So far we have already discovered the part dealing with

the fast. What remains is the how and why of nutrition which makes the Waerland diet so unique—and so effective.

Waerland appeared in London at the beginning of the Twentieth Century, to further his studies in philosophy and medicine. The young man was drawn to London by its splendid University and Library. Perhaps it was here that he could find the cause of his miserable health.

Waerland could not remember a single instant in his life when he had not been tired or weak or suffering from something or other. He always had headaches, could not concentrate and was unable to study more than one hour per day.

In his frantic search, Waerland met two scientists who sealed his fate. One was known as the greatest surgeon living, Sir Arbuthnot Lane—the other an eminent biologist, Sir Arthur Keith.

What most intrigued Waerland was Lane's surgical specialty—that of completely removing the large intestine of his patients.

With amazing speed, symptoms of arthritis, gall bladder involvements, thyroid difficulties, etc. would disappear a few days after the operation. Lane's verdict: The colon is the cause of all disease—remove it and remain free of trouble.

Keith had also been convinced that the colon had become increasingly dangerous for civilized man. His explanation: Man's digestive apparatus resembles that of the apes. I also knew that apes living in the jungle have no stomach trouble. This is why I went to Africa to find out why this was so."

The investigations revealed that the intestines of the apes contained always "natural" fermentative bacteria, whereas in the human intestine bacteria of putrefaction, capable of producing poisons, often were found to be most prevalent. There, in a nut shell was the startling discovery, that invisible bacteria could act as *effective grave diggers* to the unwitting host.

Of this, Waerland declared, that his entire method was based on Keith and Lane. But the problem was approached not by surgical operation. By means of a special diet it was attempted to tame the bacteria.

Before meeting Lane and Keith, Waerland had met another important pioneer in living reform, Dr. Alexander Haig. This man had published the book, *Uric Acid in the Causation of Disease.* The doctor had been a sufferer from migraine headaches and having gotten no relief from drugs, decided to change his diet. He gave up all butcher's meat with an improvement at once becoming apparent.

Haig contended that uric acid, being a by-product of meat— invades the tissues, resulting in rheumatism, arthritis, gout, etc., topping it off generously with all types of persistent headaches. His thesis was crystal clear, cut out the meat and get rid of the disease. He stated that diet, as presently used, is often the product of a vast amount of ignorance, a hideous waste of time. When Waerland began to read Haig's book he said he developed a fever. But it was not the fever of a disease, it was the fever of a man who had discovered something: the fever, I suppose, which besets a gold seeker when, after months of suffering in a desert, he suddenly discovers a gold mine.

With strange inner conviction, Waerland positively knew that Haig's message was the very essence he was searching. Immediately, all meat consumption was stopped and he began to feel better.

Now, with the revelations of Lane and Keith, an entirely new and promising out-look in the puzzling colon—Bacteria relationship opened up to Waerland. The research now was concentrated into physiology and bacteriology to study the behavior and habits of the intestinal tract and its germs. The findings were very significant. Digestion of ingested food in stomach, duodenum and small intestine is carried out by certain hormones and secretion manufactured in the lining of these organs. Also, digestive juices are prepared in the liver and pancreas. Thus, digestion in small intestine is afforded by chemical means.

In stark contrast to this is the colon. There, the final process of digestion is carried out by bacteria. For this reason, the colon is often referred to as the second stomach, in which the fibrous parts of the semi-liquid content is treated by the fermentative type of germs to give off its nutrients.

Here Waerland found the answer to the problem. Flesh protein, being richly associated with putrifactive bacteria, interfere or get the upper hand in the colon. With the ideal climate in the "gut" for proliferation, the bacteria multiply at a terrific rate, crowding out the friendy germs and generating a virulous poison. This is the substance that not only causes the headaches, but every conceivable malady in the body.

Waerland's suspicions of having found the real cause of his deplorable condition in the past was corroborated by many eminent authorities. It was again Lane who said that he never saw a case of cancer of the breast or female reproductive organs without the associated sorry colon putrefaction.

Waerland was convinced that by a complete turn-about in his eating habits, he could overcome all of his trouble. He had been influenced by his own experiences in isolated villages in the northern part of Sweden. There were old men of eighty and ninety—still hale and hearty, with complete sets of teeth even until advanced old age. They ate whole grain, coarse rye bread, red and green cabbage, kohlrabi, turnips, red and white beets, many potatoes and soured milk.

Waerland's most outstanding innovation is the "Kruska," a combination of several whole grain kernels, specifically prepared. Complete recipe of this truly satisfying dish is found in another chapter.

At that time, Waerland was in the middle of the twenties and when he came to Germany the first time, he was 74. It was at that age, when most others retire, that he founded the far reaching reform movement.

THE OTHER GREAT PIONEER

It is strange that the Twentieth Century in Europe should create not only one but two such outstanding humanitarians, only a few years apart—one not knowing about the existence of the other. Dr. Bircher-Benner of Switzerland was the other genius who, somewhat more effective than Waerland, was able to influence the thinking of the medical profession to a revolutionary degree.

It is about seventy years ago, that the young doctor, suffering from a serious type of yellow jaundice lost all strength. To make things worse, his digestion was in such bad shape that not a single bite could be tolerated. One day, the doctor's wife sat on his bed to prepare apples for the cooking pot. Following a sudden urge, the young wife pushed a thin slice of apple between the doctor's lips. He sucked haltingly on it and against all expectations found the apple slice most delicious. Soon all slices of one whole apple were consumed. The fruit was well received and for the next several days, nothing but raw apples were eaten.

With unbelievable surprise, the doctors noted that he was getting well and his delicate organism responded favorably to the simple food, now tasting delicious.

Soon after his recovery, Bircher-Benner was called to a woman, who had been treated without success for an advanced chronic stomach disorder by many doctors. The lady was getting progressively worse, the case appeared hopeless.

The year then was 1895, and an ironclad dictum proclaimed the teachings of the famous Max Rubner of Berlin undisputable dietary directives. This rigid indoctrination culminated in the significant factors of nutrients being provided in well cooked animal protein, fats and carbohydrates.

Since everything else so far tried had failed, and since our good doctor had cured himself by this incredible simple fare, he dared to make the attempt of treating this sinking case with a diet of raw fruit and vegetables. To the great amazement of both patient and doctor, the lady quickly improved and soon totally recovered.

Dr. Bircher-Benner was amazed and dumbfounded. He wrote: "The vegetarian had triumphed, had taught the physician a lesson."

The doctor suspected that an entirely new principle was here at work. Every effort was now made to trace the mysterious forces.

The absence of the customary meat and vegetable ration was not a sufficient explanation. There was left one possibility, could it be that the healing powers of the fruits and vegetables lay in their condition of being unfired?

At this stage, the now fully accepted Bircher-Benner method of nutrition was on its way with many tests and observations.

Accordingly, animal flesh foods suffer twice with deterioration, first by having consumed the energy providers for its own purpose and secondly because it had lost much force through heat while being prepared for consumption.

Henceforth, all flesh foods were entirely rejected by his method.

His subsequently established theories were centered on the sun, the source of all power on this earth. He regarded all green plants, leaves, fruits, tubers and roots *store houses of latent energy, absorbed from sunlight*. This energy, however, loses its intensity when becoming changed, by fading, heating or by fermentation.

In 1900, when Bircher-Benner presented this theory to the Zurich Association of Physicians, the doctors were unimpressed. "He has gone beyond the limit of science" was the cryptic verdict of the presiding officer.

Bircher-Benner was declared an outsider, "beneath the notice of science and scientific men."

Today, sixty-five years later, the findings of the doctor are accorded the greatest respect and admiration from all parts of the scientific world. A few years ago, The International Congress of Nutritionists picked out Dr. Bircher-Benner to posthumously receiving the Gold Medal—for having contributed most for suffering humanity.

The Bircher-Benner clinic of Zurich, Switzerland, presently enjoys and has enjoyed in the past the reputation of the most famous and respected health resort on this globe. Is it possible to calculate the number of untold thousands of unfortunates who had searched in vain for help in overcoming their miseries until they could recover by the very teachings so unstintingly given to the world by this unassuming doctor? A single case may be mentioned, that of a girl, age six, suffering since her third year from digestive disorders. Extreme pain in abdomen, swellings and diarrhea. The child became anemic and stopped growing. In one of the best clinics in Switzerland, all hope had been abandoned to save the child, in fact there was no record of any similar case at any time, surviving such a disorder.

Dr. Bircher-Benner was contacted by the mother of the child, a dentist from Riga. Would he take over the treatment of the small, stricken patient? Immediately, the doctor consented. The new emphasis in nutrition was put into effect. Fruit and vegetables, unheated, were used exclusively.

After eight months, the child gained fifteen pounds in weight and three inches in height. The remarks Bircher-Benner made after the correction, pointedly struck home: The "rawness" which had been deathly feared in the disease of the child was the factor responsible for the restoration of health. *The building stone, discarded by the builders, became the corner-stone.*

Are we reminded about Galileo, who was considered crazy by his contemporaries when he thought that the earth moves about the sun? The church pointed him out as a heretic and promptly excommunicated him.

THE PUZZLING CORN

The landing of the pilgrims in December, 1620 in what is now Plymouth, created a number of serious complications.

They not only had to experience all sorts of privations but actually were at the verge of starvation. There was no bread and they knew nothing about living on game, fish or berries.

By chance, the pilgrims found some corn which had been buried in the ground by some departing native tribe. A friendly Indian showed the intruders how to use the strange looking long ears of golden kernels.

Corn became and remained the most trustworthy food source to the early pioneers. It was easy to plant and gave rich rewards in speedy and plentiful harvests, with a delightful taste.

Up to this time, the United States remained the greatest producer of this prolific grain. Corn had also found its way into Europe where it was eagerly accepted.

CORN—FRIEND OR FOE FOR THE DIET?

After the Napoleonic Wars there appeared strange epidemics among the rural population of Italy. The disease was called, "pellagra" from "pella agra" or rough skin.

The disorder started with red and brownish spots on hands or feet. In some cases face, neck, knees or elbows were also affected. The mucous membrane of mouth and tongue became inflamed. In severe cases certain parts of the body became paralyzed or nervous disorders may have led to insanity.

This strange malady had also been observed in France, Spain and Rumania.

Was there a connection between the disease and the grain?

As *polenta* in Italy and the *tortilla* in Mexico corn had sustained life and strength in millions. In the New World it had rendered endurance to the great Indian cultures.

In the Southern United States corn served as the main fundament of food procurement to the people. There, as well as in Europe, people living on corn came down with the terrible disease. On the other hand, very little was known about pellagra in Mexico, Central or South America by the natives who predominantly use the golden grains.

What was the answer? In Italy, the physicians found as early as 1740 that pellagra affected only those among the poverty stricken population that lived exclusively on the product of the corn fields. If components of other food stuffs were added to the corn by the user, even in small amounts, vigor and well being would be the reward. Corn by itself, continually eaten over a certain period, spelled disease and death.

It was not until 1937 when Dr. Conrad Elvehjem found the missing substance needed to bring out the nutritional force of the corn. It was nicotinic acid and other members of the Vitamin B group. It was also found that nicotinic acid could be produced by the body from Tryptophan, one of the building blocks from protein which could be obtained from milk.

Pellagra could be prevented or quickly overcome by a few cents worth of this amazing substance.

What is the lesson taught by corn? Nature with its generosity of abundant supply makes no attempt of limiting our choice to a single food—regardless how nutritious. Every kind of food needs to be supplemented by definite substances found in other foods.

IS MANKIND FALLING APART PHYSICALLY?

Researchers in the history of mankind have found a steady

increasing deterioration in the skeletons of ancient tribes. From the appearance of the bony structures, it was possible to ascertain the respective degree of culture and soil condition.

From the earliest days several thousand years ago, the skeletons showed no signs of degeneration. But irresistibly, demonstrable signs of bony changes in following generations appeared, such as tooth decay and arthritis.

Why this downward trend? Was it physically, morally, or spiritually induced?

While it is known today that there rarely exists a singular cause, the physical, that is the respective state of soil condition must first be considered. Possibly adverse climatic changes or worn out (mined) soils no longer could provide balanced substance. The resulting nutritional deficiencies then were the direct or primary cause of the degeneration.

So much for the past. What about the present generation? How about insidious changes taking place in our bodies right now?

Not so long ago, while attending a Congress of International Nutritionists in Europe, alarming attention was called to this problem. "It is much later than we think," we were told, "look East and calculate the immensity of over-powering potential and then glance to the West and see its negative counterpart."

To grasp the true impact of this frightening statement we should be told that the speakers were no over zealous prophets, cultists or misguided "do gooders" but highly trained medical doctors, University Professors or Bio-chemists. The members of this organization are considered leaders of the profession coming from sixty-two countries all over the world, several of whom are Nobel Prize winners.

The fearful pointing to the East had nothing to do with politics, "sputniks," missiles, hydrogen bombs or things of that sort. What the statement referred to was the steady decline of the Western races in physical prowess.

It is said that the general health status of a race is in direct proportion to that of their general tooth structure. Let us look around and see how many healthy sets of teeth we can discover. Among adults it is practically impossible to find a single set free of impending decay. This deterioration of the hard mouth structures is associated with shrinkage of the gums, often leading to pyorrhea.

At this point let us establish one truism. The sorry picture of Western dental decline has nothing to do with the tooth-brush. The prevention of tooth decay by brushing or the use of mouth washes or pastes does not touch the root of the trouble. The real cause of caries does not lie on the outside but comes from within.

The curse of civilization—modern food refinement—is the chief offender. In addition any deviation in living or eating pattern interfering with a harmonious degree of body metabolism contributes to the decay found in our buccal cavities.

A great American scientist, Weston A. Price, became concerned about the problem. With an extensive dental practice in Cleveland, he had presented many papers showing the connection between bad teeth and bad food.

Dr. Price became tired of trying to remove a symptom by treating sick teeth from the outside. At the age of sixty, with great enthusiasm, the dentist-explorer went around the world. On planes, ships and by car, on horseback and on foot, the untiring gatherer of facts amassed a tremendous amount of information in the actual cause of tooth decay.

The evidence was shocking but irrefutable.

Isolated tribes were visited where all members had perfectly sound mouth structures. As long as the tribe would continue with their established eating and living pattern, there would be no tooth problem—with even the oldest members having full sets of teeth with barely a single cavity.

If, on the other hand, the tribe should establish contact with the white man with his white sugar, flour, alcohol and other civilized "blessings," the once sturdy and sound tooth structures would quickly change and decay.

Dr. Price traveled the whole length of America, from Alaska down to Peru. With almost fanatical persistency the research was continued in isolated parts of Africa and Europe.

With monotonous repetition all findings were identical. The general tooth condition of races or tribes were found to be in direct proportion to proximity or degree of contact with West-ernized food habits.

The closer to the large cities, the worse teeth and all sorts of body disorders–the more primitive and isolated–the better the teeth and greater general health.

There was not a single toothbrush found by Dr. Price, when-ever he found the enviable sets of glistening, white and pearly teeth of primitives.

A similar orientation in the tooth problem to that of Price was entertained by the German scientist Carl Roese. A physi-cian and former University Professor, Roese made investiga-tions on nearly a quarter million people, on different foods and drinking waters.

One of the continent's largest toothpaste manufacturers em-ployed the doctor to head its hygienic research department.

With truly academic thoroughness, Roese recognized the connection between tooth decay and nutrition. With total disregard to conflicting interests, the honest department chief rejected the use of the toothbrush and bacteria–destroying mouth washes. Instead, it was advised by the hygienic expert to chew a carrot or apple after each meal, providing cleansing, exercise and correct nutrition all at the same time.

As can be expected, the perplexed toothpaste manufacturer quickly corrected the situation, the over conscientious doctor was promptly fired.

THE PROTEIN ARGUMENT

How much protein does man require per day? The German investigator Carl von Voit, established an amount of 118 grams per day.

The American Atwater, Voit's student, brought the new teaching to the United States. Atwater raised Voit's quota to 145 grams.

Dr. Henry Chittenden, professor at Yale, strongly opposed Atwater as to the amounts. Chittenden came to the new con-clusions of less protein amounts by experiences gathered in his own body.

The Yale professor of chemistry suffered from arthritis, gall bladder attacks and persistent headaches. *From the 145 gram quota, Chittenden reduced the intake to barely 40 grams of protein per day. Also, he nearly cut out all flesh foods.*

The result of this food reform was most surprising. Arthritis disappeared, there were no more headaches and the gall bladder gave no more trouble.

Not only did Chittenden feel better all around, but his intellectual capacities were greatly improved. He now was firmly convinced that the customary American diet was wrong. There were too many calories and too much protein.

Experiments were now carried out under strict scientific control over a period of several years. His co-workers, students and soldiers followed faithfully the prescribed reduced diet.

The results were exactly identical with Chittenden's experiences. Everyone agreed they felt better physically and mentally.

THE MEAT PROBLEM

The principle argument in favor of meat eating is that animal protein is essential in human nutrition.

This cryptic statement not only is erroneous but has caused untold miseries to the imbibers. The slaughter of millions of animals every year for human food is unnecessary, cruel and wasteful.

It is true that meat has a stimulating effect, but this is largely due to the amounts of waste products it contains. Our nervous system can equally be stimulated by a number of poisonous substances resembling those in meat, caffeine, theobromin or nicotin, but this stimulation does not add anything to our nerve power. Muscle meat is not even a complete protein, missing are three amino-acids.

The Eskimos, living largely on meat and fat, age rapidly with a living span of but average 27½ years.

During the Czarist time, the Kirgise, a nomadic Eastern Russian tribe, were living predominantly on horse meat. The result: People matured early and equally died early. Men and women rarely passed the age of forty. The condition became so apparent, that the prevailing government attempted to change the eating habit of this wandering tribe.

What Happens on a Meat Protein Diet?

Why this advanced aging, and why does the human machinery appear to fall apart with a high meat consume? Here are the reasons:

1. Muscle meat, similar to white flour or sugar, is an incomplete food, lacking, as mentioned before, several amino-acids, as well as certain vitamins and minerals.

2. While muscle flesh does contain valuable protein, this substance is provided in great excess as required for human nutrition. *Mothers' milk contains but seven percent protein adequately furnishing not only maintenance but equally growth in the most active development period of human life.*

Let us calculate the protein percentage in our own food. Remember, if we are grown-up, the growth implication may not be considered—only maintenance. How far above the seven percent have we permitted the protein portions to out-balance the total food intake?

All responsible nutrition experts agree that protein excess disorganizes metabolism. One of its by-products is uric acid— which tends to invade many regions of the body and frequently undergoes crystallization. Gout is one symptom of such inprecipitation.

3. Animal flesh contains the waste products of the killed animal, which are poisonous. One of these substances is Xantin, closely related to the alkaloids contained in coffee and tobacco.

4. Muscle meat as such is of little taste and must therefore be prepared by cooking, frying, salting or spicing. No animal could be induced to consume such salted or spiced fare.

5. Animal flesh, fish and eggs have one thing in common, that of their rapid decomposition and putrefaction. This process generates virulent poisons predominantly in the colon. Here we find one of the main causes of constipation associated with the offensive odor of stools.

The reason for this can be found in the enormous amount of putrefactive bacteria contained in the animal fare. There are not less than 1,500,000 such decay producing bacteria in one gram of beef steak, 2,900,000 in pork, 31,000,000 in beef liver, in ground beef 75,000,000 and pork liver 95,000,000. Strangely, one gram of fish contains even more, 125 million. Still more surprising is the incredibly high amount of putrefactive bacteria contained in several day old eggs. The germs are not only putrefactive but equally pathogenic (disease causing).

Meat wears out the intestinal tract and kidneys prematurely by increasing the acidity of the blood and by accumulation of toxins in the tissues. High meat consumption favors the production of hardening of vessels—heart failure, stroke, kidney disease and cancer.

FACING THE SALT PROBLEM

Much has been said on this controversial subject. One thing is certain, civilized man takes too much of table salt or sodium chloride. What was mentioned above about frequency in urination may equally be attributed to the salt intake. Meat is tasteless without it and the resulting increasing amounts of ingested salt may be more responsible for urinary derangement than the meat itself.

The European research about the salt question revealed that the kidneys could cope with eliminating up to five grams per day. Any amount above that somehow has to be tolerated by the system. The splitting of the salt into sodium and chlorine could ease the situation, particularly when up to twenty-five grams of salt are taken daily.

There is no question that salt hardens tissues. The medical expert is in full agreement to that, this is the reason why he forbids the use of salt in serious cases of heart, vessel or kidney involvement.

It is entirely possible to get along nicely without the use of salt, particularly so if the flesh consumed is abandoned. All the salts needed by the body are plentifully supplied by fruits and vegetables.

However, small amounts of salt may improve the taste of some foods. In our home we use exclusively sea salt extracted without heat. Surprisingly a little will go far—incidentally doing their part to the balancing of minerals in the body.

THE NEW VEGETARIAN CONCEPT

There were people already 2500 years ago, who discovered the healing force of living food. Pythagoras, the "originator of Science," taught that only "living fresh" foods could enable man to "apprehend the truth."

Perhaps in this statement we find the explanation in the ambiguities involved with the term vegetarianism. The meat eaters often point out the undeniable fact that there are sick vegetarians. Waerland called these meat abstainers "Pudding Vegetarians filling themselves with over cooked refined carbohydrates."

The impact of the new evaluation was to recognize the difference between "live" and dead foods. Live foods denoting fruits, seeds, vegetables, in fact any edible plant, root, fruit, berry *unchanged* by man. "Dead foods" referring to animal flesh, eggs, fish and all the products of the soil changed by man through refining or subjections to heat.

PITFALLS OF MODERN FOOD PROCESSING METHODS

A few thoughts should be added about modern food processing methods resulting in more untimely deaths and crippling of unwitting victims than were suffered by all wars in the history of mankind.

Radio and Television have become the accepted entertainment medium for the masses. This powerful vehicle is cleverly used to condition the mass mind to the use of products with a wide margin of profits. After all, someone has to pay for the "circus" so eagerly demanded by the masses. Pain pills and laxatives fitted nicely into the picture as can be attested by the choice selections of programs supported by these commodities. Cigarette advertising also assumes a generous slice of the entertainment budget. Yet, there is still more room for others.

The Madison hucksters were able to convince the food refiners about certain psychological implications of repetition.

By establishing a conformity pattern, the food processors were able to sell their products at enormous profits.

To get an idea as to the scope of these profits, just ask any farmer how much he gets from the millers for his grain. You may be astounded to learn about the difference there exists between the growers' reward and the price tag attached to the finished product. The breakfast cereals with their phony claims clearly establish the point.

The tragedy of the situation lies not so much in the inflated price structures of the products, but taking over perfectly nutritious food and rendering it fit for ornaments on the shelves of super-markets. The incidental *change of live foods by the trickeries of the chemist into lifeless substances resembling wall paper paste, is of grave concern.*

It is only fair to include that the food processors, by the very nature of their business, have no choice to do otherwise.

Their only alternative for reform would be to get out of the processing business entirely and limit activities solely to the packaging of whole grains or other whole foods. This would involve the assessments of re-educational practices in all segments of populations. Also who would pay What to Whom to carry out the task? And in the meantime, how about the circus on the screen, which by now the masses fully expect to be carried on and on?

It is generally known that the refinement of cereals removes the outer layer including most minerals and vitamins. A recently discovered substance is also lost, known as "auxone." This mysterious living force, exceedingly small, is able to provoke the manufacture of vitamins in the human digestive organs. How tragic, the single loss of this infinitesimal substance precludes the "seeding" of our "intestinal gardens." The amount of this "home produced" vitamin is enough to stagger the imagination, said to be from *three to fifty times* the usual amounts taken with our food.

It has been learned that the Auxones play an important part in the replacement and rejuvenation of body cells.

The question may be asked, how is it possible that the human machine can continue to operate in view of all aforementioned food deficiencies or other nutritional inconsistencies?

The answer is that providence possibly foresaw such a contingency and equipped the human organism with certain faculties to replenish elements missing in some foods by appropriation from other foods. This is possibly the reason why the prevalence of scurvy, beriberi or pellagra is rarely seen in epidemic proportions in our country even though such disease can often be detected in borderline degrees.

Many times the potato has helped to prevent the total collapse of some individuals. In extreme cases, life will go on, if only some Vitamin B-1, a few minerals and a little protein is supplied to the organism.

There exists an amazing ability in the human machine to adapt itself to adverse conditions and thus permit the living process to carry on.

A state of "half health" is maintained by a large number of unwitting performers in this great drama of food, habits and life.

The Peckham experiment revealed interesting data about this state of half health. Bircher-Benner termed it "pregnant health" and McCollum called it the "twilight zone of disease" produced by a diet on which no race in history has ever yet attempted to live.

The nutritional experiment was significant in that a group of middle class people participated, not rich nor poor, who, from all appearances were considered normally healthy. There were 4,000 members of the Peckham Health Center of London, England, carefully studied over a period of nine years. All members of the group belonged to the "best" age consideration, between 20 and 42.

The incredible result: *Ninety-one percent were sick and only nine percent healthy.* Most everyone then had been afflicted with defect of glands, heart, kidney or other organs, clinically detectable. Of these, only one quarter of the sick felt that there was something wrong with them. The other three-quarters were stunned to learn about the objective findings. In some cases, they even displayed signs of exuberant health, when the existence of serious disorders had been established.

Of the one-quarter sick who "knew" about their disorders, only one-third did something about it by consulting a doctor. The others tried to get along as best as possible, only searching for help when unable to do so.

Of the nine percent, who were considered "healthy" all were males in their twenties. The fact that discernible diseases could not be diagnosed did not mean that the men possessed a high degree of vitality. In no way could they compare to the Hunzas or other vital races when considering stamina and physical exuberance.

A true diagnostic condition could be established only after death, in post-mortems. Out of the Korean conflict, such an evaluation received alarming attention by all health authorities. There were two-hundred young American soldiers, with an average age of twenty-two years, who were killed in action. The examination revealed that seventy-seven and three-tenths percent had gross evidence of hardened vessels in heart. If we take these figures as an average, we must conclude that three-quarters of the young men today or soon will have the potentials of coronary thrombosis.

The young men belonged to a nation having the highest scientific development. There followed an examination of a similar number of oriental counterparts in the same age group, in action. The results were astounding, the presence of heart abnormalities was practically non-existant.

Returning to the Peckham experiment, the results are crystal clear. Less than one-tenth of all people examined were free of disease, as can be determined in the living body. Considering the somewhat dubious health distinction of this group as indicated above, it is more shocking to learn about the true detectable disorders in the other nine-tenths.

In this country, at the University hospital, Ann Arbor, Michigan, five-hundred apparently healthy business men were examined. Their average age was forty-eight years. Nearly half of them suffered from physical disease of which they were not aware, requiring immediate treatment.

In another study at the University of Pennsylvania, of one thousand apparently healthy individuals, only thirteen percent were found entirely free of defects.

5

The Law of Wholeness of Foods

All natural foods, fruits, seeds (nuts), vegetables, roots, etc. are combinations of certain elements. These components are proteins, carbo-hydrates, fats, minerals, vitamins, auxones, enzymes, etc. Complete utilization of the foods can only take place in the presence of all of these elements.

For the purpose of maintaining preservation, all nutritious objects have been equipped by nature with a protective covering, to permit food provisions to carry over a period of scarcity or into the next season. In the case of grass seeds (cereals) this protective mechanism is so perfect as to allow the grains to survive untold years of storage.

Tombs in Egypt have revealed containers filled with grain kernels, "stored" several thousand years ago. It was found that the cereals, while exceedingly hard and brittle, under subjection to moisture began to sprout. The inherent life force, imperative for sound nutrition, had been kept intact.

The law of wholeness also takes into account the fact that *all* food factors must be present if optimum nutrition is to be attained. The taking of a single supplement therefore often is not the entire solution of the food problem. As pertaining to vitamins, the entire chain in a formula should be considered. Minerals and trace elements can be obtained from the sea, in the form of kelp or dulse.

The peelings of fruits should not be discarded, nor the seeds or structures surrounding it. Most important nutritional components are found there. The apple is an example. The core, including seeds, contains twenty times as much iodine and other minerals as the whole of the rest of the apple. This fact should be significant in view of the increasing prevalence of thyroid symptoms.

Waerlands' phenomenal success, in converting large segments of European populations to a healthful diet, above all, is based on the concept of wholeness of foods.

Grains were chosen, because of their availabilities in all seasons in all parts of the world. The grain kernels had to be intact and several varieties were recommended to forestall deficiencies of elements lacking in the single type.

The grain dish, known as Kruska was immediately prepared and eaten after the grain had been reduced to a grit by a mixer or small mill. The contact of air (oxygen) would reduce the live force of the cereals in a matter of days.

The rule: Mill or grind only enough grains needed for intended meal, keep supply in dry container.

UNFIRED (RAW) FOODS

There is no doubt that the art of cookery has brought about certain enrichments to our table. Heat destroys bacteria and parasites such as worm eggs and trichinas which attach themselves to food. Even until a short while ago, it was believed that only through heat could the vegetable be appropriated as food, as the cooking would burst the membrane of the vegetable cell. This long prevailing assumption has been found to be erroneous. Unheated vegetable cells are successfully worked upon by the digestive juices, as is the case with boiled ones.

I fully agree with the heat indoctrination when it comes to protect the body from harmful bacteria and parasites. These organisms do constitute a serious problem for the meat eater. Since it is the purpose of this book to discourage the use of all animal flesh foods, we may disregard this provision.

The customary cooking of leaf, root or other vegetables destroys the greater part of the electro-magnetic force, stored by the sun. This destruction starts even at relatively low temperatures of 140° F. and becomes more serious the longer the cooking lasts. Spinach, or cabbage, as an example, cooked in the customary way, retains only one fortieth part of its original food content.

What an incredible, sad loss. Just ponder and think, one must eat forty times the amount of plant foods prepared the old way, as against eating the substance unheated. This explains why only comparatively small amounts of the raw variety is sufficient to satisfy the "cravings" for food.

Dr. Ziegelmeyer, a bio-chemist, made these assertions about this important problem: Raw food secures the keeping of *"key" food substances*, prevents the denaturing of proteins. Cooking interferes with high molecular combinations, changes surface and osmotic tension and reduces the energy potential."

Kollath states: "Let the natural be as natural as possible."

There are a few excellent foods which seem to withstand the changes incurred by heat. One is the potato, which surprisingly keeps its nutritive excellence when cooked or baked. The beautiful, healthy and vigorous Irish women certainly prove this point. But, remember, no peeling, no water insertion. Potato is *steamed* or baked in jacket, and as such consumed.

CONSTANT FOOD CRAVINGS

How many times does the doctor hear this complaint of heat-treated foods. Nutrition experts have always diagnosed this condition as "mineral starvation" which doubtless it is. But the core of the matter goes deeper. Not only minerals are starving but all the other life forces held together by the *mysterious cosmic energy* so generously given by the sun to the plant. This force is to be temporarily stored for the purpose of creating and maintaining life on this planet.

Over-cooking, refining, denaturing, makes food lifeless, the fuel to the human machinery has become counterfeit. The products from the bakery greatly contribute along these lines, since three of the most widely tampered-with eating substances are involved. White sugar, white flour, and hydrogenated fat, plus innumerable synthetic chemicals are the culprits enjoying the number one position in the make-up of *food-less* foods.

How to Overcome Craving for Food

Constant food cravings can be overcome in a matter of a few weeks or even days. A total fast of three to seven days should start the change to be followed with Kruska—raw salad —baked or steamed potato diet, eating sparingly and well chewed. Remember all implication of the colon. Get rid of all decay producing bacteria by omitting animal flesh, fish or even eggs. One or two slightly steamed vegetables could be included for those of greatly impaired digestion. Even this small amount of heat application should be reduced or entirely ignored. Putrefactive bacteria, responsible for most systemic disorders, are counteracted by lactic acid. Good sources are yogurt, sour milk, buttermilk, cottage cheese, sauerkraut and sour pickles.

You may counter that such a simple diet could provide little in the culinary pleasures we expect to enjoy on the table. In this thought you have plenty of company. In my own case, I repeatedly had rejected such a "poor man" fare as being "inconsistent to social status." Is it not true that sometimes we cannot see the trees for the forest?

Could it be a wise province of the universe to subject man to all kinds of temptations to have him prove his worth? Is it not food which dominates the chief urge of man—that of self preservation? Does there exist a definite purpose in the universe of permitting the "beclouding" of man in order for him to rise above it and establish his admittance to the inner circle of "initiates"? "The survival of the fittest" may not only be limited to biological meanings in high school classrooms, but also assumes deeper significances in the emancipation of the human mind. Mental and spiritual developments are contingent upon the physical framework. A continuous chain reaction is at work. The nutrition problem, with its temptation lure, is used by Providence to make the selection.

How strange, the simple but natural foods awaken a long forgotten sensation of taste delight. Also, what is amazing is the exceedingly small amounts of food intake we now find generally satisfactory. Surprisingly, one can get along on much less than formerly accustomed to. An average of fifty grams of protein daily will be generally sufficient to keep us in the "pink" of condition. The rest of the food can also be reduced, in many cases to half the former amount.

There still will be many skeptics who will find the above deductions incredible and fantastic. I can fully understand their doubts, as I once was one of them. I am not asking them to change their mind but afford me the simple courtesy of a trial. *It was Ruskin who said: "A single grain of solid fact is worth ten tons of theory."*

There is no need to extend the trial period over months or years. Two weeks, or even only ten days will establish the truth of this new behavior and eating pattern. A few days' food fast followed with the suggested diet in chapters following will definitely convince the most dubious about the superiority of this concept. Remember also, it is not always the price tag which determines the quality of the product.

An old axiom expresses this succinctly: "The higher the price of the meal—the less the health benefits to the body."

THE SUGAR EATING PROBLEM

We are now concerned with white sugar, coming from sugar cane, or beets. The fantastic amounts consumed by the American people are shocking to those having an inkling of biochemistry.

McCann has demonstrated the solubility of calcium in water, the relationship being one part of calcium to 1000 parts of water. Sugar has an affinity for calcium and if added to the water, the amount of dissolved calcium is *thirty-five times as much.* Is it any wonder that it is almost impossible to find a single healthy set of teeth here in the "best fed" nation on earth? And yet, the prevailing cult is to scrub the teeth *from the outside,* without much regard to the fantastically high consuming of leeching *white sugar,* one of the curses of civilization.

Sugar, the ultra-refined sweet, in the refining process has practically every health element removed, the remaining white substance resembling carbon. Assimilation of any food substances can take place only in the presence of certain elements known as "catalysts." Since these supporting live elements have been removed, the needed substances must be withdrawn from the body structures, wherever available. Teeth, bones and glands are normally richly supplied with these elements but slowly and surely the body supply dwindles, with beginning signs of degeneration in various parts of the body.

In the order of frequencies, the teeth become the first victim of the disturbed body chemistry. The endocrine (ductless) glands follow next with the bony segments (skeleton) and remaining tissues not far behind in catching up with the others.

How Sugar Attacks You

From a bio-chemical view, the sugar disturbs the calcium-phosphorous relationship, caused by the leaching of body structures. Of course, a part of the blame should also be accorded to white flour, in fact to any grain product subjected to refinement by the chemist in food production.

The pulp, dentin and—surprise—even the enamel becomes attacked within from the lymph stream to apprehend substances critically in demand at the time. Poor Mama, she suspects junior not to be too consistent with the toothbrush. Perhaps, the deadly germs must be met not only once—but after each meal? Does the unsuspecting parent understand that the brushings could have possible abrasive actions on the outer enamel of teeth, more valid in view of the disturbed body chemistry?

The Carbohydrate Villain

As pertaining to the endocrine glands, the telltale effects of the one-sided carbohydrate intake does not take much time to become noticeable. The thyroid becomes involved with erratic functions. Secretions become too much, or too little. Over secretions may lead to protruding eyes, under production to obesity.

In the pancreas we find microscopic specks bunched together, the size of pin heads. These small separated structures are called Islands of Langerhans, named after their discoverer. Their purpose is the manufacture of insulin, essential in the utilization of starches and sugar. The evil of refinements un-relentingly marches on. The raw materials required to concoct the secretion are no longer available in sufficient amounts. The production of insulin is greatly reduced or stopped entirely. Diabetes has arrived!

This dreadful disease is prevalent in direct proportion to the intake of both white sugar and flour. Diabetes was practically unknown before the appearance of the food refinement cult. The number of its victims can be calculated with astounding accuracy by the respective consumption of the unbalanced product.

Superimposed upon the thyroid gland we find little bodies the size of peas, known as the para-thyroid glands. Their function: to regulate the use of calcium in the body. As we have seen above, the robbing of essentials for the production of its specific secretion is equally carried on by the lymph stream with ruthless efficiency from the small but so important regulators. The show must go on, in spite of overpowering odds in the lack of life maintaining components. Death must be cheated —even at the expense of permitting only flickers of the subdued flame of life.

Arthritis is on the march, approaching in giant strides. Joints become painful and the poor victim is advised that there is no cure and that aspirin affords the only relief.

In some individuals, the disturbed calcium chemistry affects muscles and tendons. We speak now of rheumatism or the "misery" so pointedly and colloquially expressed in the South. It could practically be the same thing with the exception of cases where intakes of insufficiently cooked pork brings on the pain. A parasitic involvement is here the contributory cause, rarely the sole one. The trichina enters the muscle tissues, encapsulates itself and through pressure or other irritations to the sensory nerves creates the aches, the condition known as trichinosis.

Returning to sweets, another interesting problem has been connected to the eating of *refined carbohydrates*, particularly sugar. In all Westernized countries, people are growing taller with decided changes in structure and sizes of the bony frame. In America, as an example, children of immigrants coming from Europe are one to two inches taller than their parents. The following generation seems to perpetuate this direction of increased growth by becoming still taller.

The feet absorb a generous share of this tendency toward bigness. It is even suspected that the size increase of the feet is out of proportion to the rest of the body. Recently, an ungallant story made the rounds, commenting about the heroic efforts required by the chivalrous escort to down the drink in his lady's slipper. It is difficult for the American tourist to buy shoes in South America or Asia. The larger sizes are simply not available.

The increase of length to the bones brings more serious consequences in other regions. In the hip, the bones become longer in length—but shorter in width. The female pelvis becomes slimmer, explaining the increasing difficulties encountered in childbirth.

Not so long ago, a test was made in which alarming indications of this bone-change phenomenon were noted. Several boys and girls of high school age were placed against the wall, with their backs exposed, but heads covered up.

The examining doctors could not tell which was what—there was not the slightest clue observed in the bodies pointing to male or female characteristics.

The Mal-Effects of Sugar

The Japanese nutrition expert, Dr. A. Katase, made painstaking experiments on animals over a period of ten years. The subject: Effects of refined sugar in growth, development and behavior of animals.

The findings were frightening. *The bone structure became deranged*, the long bones became longer, with similar narrowings of pelvic shapes as observed in the high school examination.

Still more damaging was the test's revelation on composition of bones. The emphasis always was degenerations in a more or less degree. A decided softening of the bones was noted, in some cases bones being so soft that they could be scraped easily with a knife blade.

Dr. Katase proved that the organism could accommodate a *small amount of refined sugar,* conditioned by the liver into glycogen. Any *additional* amount is immediately absorbed by osmosis into the circulation, to be converted to free carbonic acid. To keep the organism free of the corrosive action of this acid, calcium had been withdrawn from the bones for neutralization. Hand in hand with this development went the enlargement and beginning degeneration of the parathyroid glands, the little pea shaped specks located in front of the thyroid.

The calcium has to be leached (settled) out of the bones to control the over-acidity of the fluids and soft tissues. The disposition of the extracted lime salts now assumes critical proportions. The material has to be shelved somewhere, conditions permitting. Calcium carbonate, ruthlessly evicted from its household, precipitates into the soft meshes of muscles, tissues and—vessels. Slowly but unerringly, blood and lymph vessels become coated or permeated with the cementing agent. Arterosclerosis, hardening and brittleness of vessels is underway! Arteries may easily burst; if damage occurs in brain, we will have stroke; in heart, a coronary occlusion.

The amount of refined sugar which *could* be tolerated by the human organism has been estimated to be less than twenty grams per day for an adult. For a child weighing forty pounds the respective amount would be six grams, in the infant one gram per day.

The far reaching impact of these figures can be summarized when we consider the actual consumption of white sugar. The per capita amount being over one-hundred pounds annually puts the daily use at about one-hundred-fifty grams. The safety limits have been and still are being disregarded seven and one-half times.

So much for Katase's findings and suggested reform. Our own stand on the problem is a little simpler.

What *is* our answer? To any thinking person, there is but one. It spells DON'T. Do not use it. By all means quit this very minute eating anything on your shelf that is not natural food. Do not give it away, not even to your enemy. Remember, refined foods, given to animals, will always respond in degeneration and death. Is it so difficult not to expect the same in man?

GLUCOSE, THE ARCH ENEMY

It is almost impossible to think that there could be other commodities, still worse than white sugar. There is, a more synthetic sweet, made out of corn starch, treated with sulphuric acid.

On super market shelves all sorts of bright colored candies, jellies, jams, etc. beckon to be taken home. While some of these concoctions may contain natural food products, the sugary parts may be the glucose variety.

A leading diabetic authority, stated that owing to the present trend of increase in diabetes, *in another fifty years the American people might all be diabetic.*

CHEMICAL SWEETS

In this category we find sacharin, dulcin, etc., deriving from a synthesis out of coal tars. The present trend of soft drinks to evade the calorie problem leads to increased use of these products.

The sugar problem can easily be solved. Use only *raw* cane or beet sugar or better yet use good old bee honey. How nourishing, and delicious! Get a jar and find out for yourself. I am sure you will be pleasantly surprised. Acquire the Kruska habit—supplemented with crisp raw salads, fresh fruits with an occasional dish of legumes (see chapters on recipes). I do not recommended coal tar derivatives for sweeteners in any food or beverage.

PLEASURES, INSTINCTIVE AND ACQUIRED

I realize in some, and many cases, it is getting pretty late. The teeth may all be gone, with the store sets giving the owner away with occasional revealing whistles. The joints no longer are as elastic as they had been and the bowels or kidneys are not doing too well either.

Will the new food trial bring back the horses, after the barn door had been kept open? The obvious answer is no, but one thing I am sure of—great—surprisingly great relief can be obtained by a religious adherence to suggestions given in this book.

Remember, the meanings of joys or pleasures are relative. The inveterate cigarette smoker may insist that he gets pleasure from smoking. But this same man will have to agree that this feeling of pleasure primarily had to be acquired. The first cigarette was everything but pleasant, but in spite of it, by conformity the habit is started. Later, the inevitable effects of drug addiction take hold and the smokers find "pleasure" in sucking the smoke containing the alkaloids.

In a similar fashion, sensations of pleasure can be cultivated from the eating of harmful foods. Think about the candy, doughnut, cake and soft drink habit, all giving relative "pleasures."

Surprisingly, animal flesh belongs in the same category of providing "pleasure." In this case it is obtained from the meat containing alkaloids, with their stimulating action. It may be shocking to some of us to learn that we are imbibing narcotics, when partaking in the eating of meat.

We have digressed somewhat to establish the meaning of pleasure. The point is knowing that there are several types. Some pleasures are deeply inherent, instinctive and satisfy constructively. Other pleasures are of *relative* significance. They later had to be learned in the over-coming of inborn natural protective instincts. This explains the sickening feeling after the first cigarette or the belching or burning signals uttered by protesting digestive organs. We could also include the resulting disgust most of us experience when passing a butcher shop. The "enjoyment" of meat is definitely a relative and learned pleasure.

What is so amazing is to discover our own immense capacities for adjustment. Once the mind has appropriated the truth, an unrelenting change in our feelings surges ahead. Natural instincts again take over, with a reshuffling of pleasure concepts.

Not all of us can benefit from such a reform, directed by our own free will. When I returned from Argentina with the evidence and pictures of Dr. Roffo's cancer experiments, showing the horrible and gory results of smoking in my professional classes, I could always expect a certain percentage of my students to quit the habit.

I mentioned a "certain percentage," why not all of them? Simply, the message did not go through, their minds refused to accept it. Remember, not all of us, only some do recognize the truth, when presented. When the pupil is ready, the master will appear.

THE UBIQUITOUS GERM OR BACTERIA

The French chemist, Louis Pasteur, discovered a number of different germs while investigating the cause of fermentation. First rejected and then eagerly accepted, the discovery of the germs now established the cause of disease. Man goes by beliefs and this bacteria supposition was tailored to order with its immense potential for commercial exploitation.

The mentality of the masses has been encouraged to maintain certain specific beliefs. No one but Waerland could express it more pointedly: "Man requires a heaven and a hell, a God and a master devil, angels and small devils, a lost paradise and a paradise to be regained."

"The microbe mania has conquered the mind of people so easily because the microbes fitted so well into an old form of belief. Microbes merely replaced the old devils."

Having spent a life time in the treatment of disease, I am positive that germs do *not* cause disease. The germs are the *results* of the disease.

Back in 1914, Dr. Rosenow, then considered America's most eminent bacteriologist, associated with the Mayo Foundation, published a most interesting paper. The results of painstaking experiments were documented. So important were the contents of this paper that it shattered the foundation of the serum and drug industry.

The findings of Rosenow verified the conclusions of Bechamp and others. It was established that there exists no specific bacteria. One kind of bacteria were changed to other kinds of bacteria and back again. How? Simply by altering condition, food and temperature of environment. *Deadly bacteria were converted to harmless ones and vice-versa.*

The Rosenow experiments show that bacteria are not of themselves deadly or dangerous, but merely a primitive form of life. The condition of the host determines the behavior of the germ, either beneficial or dangerous. If we permit our bodies to undergo changes of degeneration, if the process of putrefaction becomes apparent, the rapidly propagating germs could be termed dangerous. Even at this stage, to accuse the germ of hostility is difficult to understand. After all, the germ merely carries out its accorded duty, that of scavenging and freeing the body of decay. Where and what kind of decay, it may be asked? In the breakdown of protein by the bacteria, poisonous substances are produced. Back in 1888, Dr. Senator founded the concept of "Autointoxication," meaning self poisoning from metabolic end-products generated in the cleansing process by the germ scavengers. It was not so much the bacteria that were at fault, but the excessive protein, predominantly coming from flesh foods, fish and eggs.

If on the other hand, we live in accordance to sound nutrition and behavior principally, germs, always present, will be helpful.

As early as 1897, Dr. Lemke closely studied this problem and observed that the dietary change from meat to bread, fruits and vegetables resulted in a complete alteration in the intestinal bacteria and incidental disappearance of poisonous substances.

The famous Russian Metchnikoff created a sensation with his projection of intestinal bacteria into polite society. Having postulated the toxic implications of the putrefactive germs, he concentrated his attention on conditions that would by-pass the decay genesis.

In checking the living span of people, he found that inhabitants of Bulgaria reached the greatest age, and remained free of aches and pains, even when old. This was most challenging to the brilliant investigator and an intensive search for the cause of this exuberant health condition was soon discovered, *lactic acid as found in yogurt, sour milk and sauerkraut*. It was not Metchnikoff's fault that a one-sided emphasis on yogurt was instigated without regard to other nutritional aspects. Not only the nearly complete absence of flesh products in the diet of the Bulgarians had been ignored, but also their strict adherence to a sparse but unhampered natural fare of whole grains, fruits and vegetables.

THE FRIENDLY BACTERIA

The "good" bacteria, leaving lactic acid as their end-product, now became an object of intense study. An amazing new scope of activity was credited to these tiny little workers. It was found that they not only counteracted adverse effects of putrefaction but actually were manufacturing vitamins in the intestines. It has been proven that nine vitamins are made, among them Vitamin K and the B complex vitamins.

The bacteria work in conjunction with auxones, found in seeds and green leaves.

In 1943, two American scientists, Majjar and Holt carried on some interesting experiments. One group of young men received a carefully prepared diet containing all essential components except Vitamin B-1. After several months, there were no visible signs of Vitamin deficiencies, it was being eliminated, in spite of the fact that it was absent from the diet. This vitamin elimination stopped immediately as soon as some antibiotic remedy destroyed the intestinal bacteria.

The Munich professor Baumgaertl, a top authority on the intestinal flora, declared in 1954 that the *chemo-therapeutic treatment of many infectious diseases created drastic harm to the patients. The treatment destroyed the intestinal flora, which led to serious symptoms of vitamin deficiencies and to more dangerous intestinal infections. Antibiotics, while destroying the specific causes of the primary infection, also destroyed the vitamin producing bacteria.*

GENERAL CONSIDERATIONS FOR A
HEALTH DIET

Nearly twenty-eight years have passed since I became acquainted with this new form of life. As formerly mentioned, I had suffered a heart attack and was told to get my things in order as there was little hope of recovery.

Bernarr MacFadden got me started. The astounding results from the fast, plus the new insight into a different living pattern, completely changed my life. I had to know all there was to it, resulting in may years of study and travel.

That the fasting principle worked, I became convinced of, but what about the diet. How can one eat to keep from having trouble? The vegetarian diet did make sense to me, right at the beginning. But there were many variations in that eating concept which often left me wondering whether or not I was on the right track.

Several times I had to repeat long fasts to correct conditions obviously not prevented by the vegetarian diet.

I kept on trying and searching. Several times I returned to the meat diet only to repent quickly and return to the aesthetics of vegetarianism. All forgiven, I contemplated, rather to take into account some apparent inconsistencies and suffer silently, than to follow the crowd and re-appropriate a way of eating which nearly had succeeded in casting my doom.

In retrospect, how clearly can we identify our mistakes. What I did wrong is that which thousands of similar minded people have been and still are doing.

The emphasis of my orientation was projected into one objective, that of eliminating meat from the daily fare. Otherwise, I carried on the best I could. Cooked starchy foods and eggs became my main consideration. I developed into a *Pudding Vegetarian* as so ably expressed by Waerland.

The Raw Food Diet

When I finally realized the *destructive effects of heat upon food,* I decided to try a complete *raw food regimen* for one month. The results were electrifying, within a few days I felt much stronger with a return of my former enthusiasm. Many of my patients whom I had been able to convert to this new diet, also reported similar results.

All sorts of experiments were carried out on many patients, suffering from every conceivable ailment. Some of these tests were counter checked in my own body in order to arrive at a more scientific and generalized effect of a specific diet.

The results were always the same. The meat intake seemed to satisfy the taste and produced an apparent apprehension of well being. But a drastic change in the feeling would take over very soon. In a matter of a few hours, often less than one hour, a decided degree of fatigue was felt.

In cases of arthritic tendencies, occasional flare ups of pain in joints were noted. Microscopic examination of stool always revealed putrefactive bacteria, sometimes in such staggering amounts that all of the examined portions seemed to consist of these living and squirming organisms. In this, a significant phase had been noted. The odor of the stools had been influenced by the diet. The intake of meat always resulted in the odor becoming putrid; eliminate the meat, the odor would be less offensive.

A fantastic correlation was noticed, the appearance of aches and pains very often being in direct proportion to the degree of odoriferousness of the stools, and type of colon bacteria.

In vegetarian diets, the odor indication also became significant. The degree of heat applications or state of refinement in the fare equally responded in respective unpleasant odors. It could only be deducted that certain agents in the diet were either missing or had been altered by the heat.

The respective protein content of the vegetarian diet had also been found to be indicative of changes in the intestinal flora. Legumes such as beans, lentils, peas, etc. equally contributing to the display of putrifactive changes.

Protein Intake

Another interesting point became apparent. *The characteristics of bacteria and odor were influenced by the AMOUNT of protein. Even vegetable proteins could bring about autointoxication to the patient if used in excess* as evidenced by the bacteria and stool.

What can we learn from this experiment? First that the purpose of the bacteria in the large intestine is to break down cellulose and hard fibers, being a part of seeds and plants or fruits. The bacteria converts sugars and starches into lactic acid, which in turn acts to neutralize poisonous end-products generated in the digestion of proteins by the same germs. This neutralization principle operates *effectively only if the percentage of the protein in the food fare is held to the right amount.* The mother's milk index of seven percent could be taken as a guide. Since this protein percentage is to provide food components in a period of most rapid human growth development, it is safe to assume that even this low percentage could be reduced in the diet of grown-ups.

So far we have considered vegetarian protein. As soon as animal flesh is substituted or added, the problem of bacteria disorientation immediately becomes increasingly more acute.

Even if the percentage relationship is held within the lower amounts, bacteria and stool characteristics tend to gravitate into the field of putrefaction.

Plant and Meat Proteins

So far, I have not been able to find out all the reasons why the untiring little colon germs should take such a hostile attitude against flesh proteins. Here we find one of the most intriguing puzzles in the nutritional field and further research is needed. At any rate, we know that there is a difference between vegetable and flesh protein, as there is between the cooked or uncooked variety.

The formerly discussed auxones, missing in meat, may partially explain the problem. Foods rich in auxones are seeds, sour milk, yougurt, green leaves and tubers. The protein of the potato is said to be of highest nutritional quality, even when cooked or baked. What it all boils down to is for us to repent and become impressed by the old story of naturalness.

The human cell is composed of molecules, which in turn are made out of atoms put together by electrons. Putting it in a more crude term, we are essentially a composition of billions of electrical units, being both generators and motors. The human electro-chemical engine is sustained with powers coming from the sun. The vegetable cover of the earth—that is all green plants with their fruits are repositories of the sun's energy. No life then can exist without extracting it out of the plants, either primarily or secondarily. In the latter case, the plant products had been converted to animal flesh, to act as temporary storehouses. In rivers, lakes or oceans, sea life also follows a similar pattern, only in addition to plants, certain small organisms such as algae, plankton, etc. serve as storage facilities.

The human organism is constructed in such a way to most efficiently utilize the sun's energy made available in its primary form, as stored in the plant kingdom. This does not mean that the secondary stored force of the sun could not support life—it can—but, as the term implies, it can do only second best.

The bacteria is equally dependent for its existence upon the energy derived from the sun. Its living purpose, that of breaking down, converting and extracting nutrients, must be geared to the exact requirement of substances it is called to work upon.

The bacteria, in its optimal performance, leaves lactic acid as the end-product, guaranteeing vitality to the host. *The increased protein intake, even from vegetable source, will result in an inverse ratio of germ efficiency.*

Imperturbably, the approach of decay is in sight. In the case of animal protein, a more sinister bacterial change can be expected. The production of lactic acid no longer is sufficient to neutralize the increasing amounts of poisonous left overs in the protein conversion. The bacteria is forced to change its structure and behavior to meet or counteract the new situation. In many cases, the required task is so stupendous, as to over tax the ability of even this now altered aggressive germ. The upshot is putrefaction.

The bacteria now becomes more prolific—it reproduces at an incredible rate to literally devour the opponent. Over three quarters of the intestinal mass may thus become "alive," it actually moves on the slide of the miscroscope.

Now we are coming to the heart of the matter. Protein is a most useful and important part of food. To be without it would spell death, to have too much, bring discord and disease. Anyone with open eyes can see the result of the presently stylish protein mania, followed practically everywhere.

But let us follow the decay processes, originating in the

colon. The germ, like all living things, takes in food, digests it and gives off its waste. When it attacks protein, it comes in contact with highly complex substances in the process of digestion. These materials belong in the category of alkaloids and somewhat resemble opiates in their effects upon nerve tissues. This explains partially the cause of "spastic colon," where the muscular wall of the intestine is held by continued contractions. X-ray examinations often have revealed this grip-like squeeze to reduce the size of lumen (diameter) of the tube to that of a pencil. The accumulating poisons must be removed at all costs. In some cases the body resorts to occasional attacks of diarrhea, a forceful flushing of the bowel.

The Lymph Filters

But certain amounts of the poisons are absorbed by the blood stream. The lymph nodes become aroused to action. By a process of filtering, they try to keep the blood free of harmful ingredients. To cope with the increased demand, they become enlarged and frequently clogged with filtered waste, which it had been unable to neutralize by specific secretions and cells (lymphocites). The glands become enlarged and painful. Mechanical removal of these protecting devices is often resorted to, as evidenced by appendix and tonsil surgery.

The overwork or crippling of the lymphatic system permits the spilling over of poisons into the general circulation. The next protective mechanism goes into action. The liver, spleen and adrenals try to do their best, in detoxifying the blood. This over taxing effort may be carried out over many years, occasionally interrupted by fatigue symptoms of this heroic defensive force.

With the increased demand, the organs often enlarge, but invariably break down. A dangerous situation has arisen. The glands not only have commenced to be less effective in keeping the body free from poisonous substances, they themselves become attacked by the waste products. Degeneration sets in, in its varied manifestations. The kidneys, last bastion of defense, had to put in overtime work practically from the start.

The urinary apparatus goes out of gear. With its filtering purpose defaulting, metabolic end-products are permitted to become deposited in tissues, under, over, around and inside of cells. Often, the offending material changes into crystals, interfering with nerve passage, and circulation. Local symptoms are pressure and aches and pain.

Bacterial Breakdown

Such can be the result of the spread of toxins generated in the large intestine. But more complicating, the bacteria themselves can wander away from their operating field and invade distant regions. The small intestine, normally separated by a valve from the colon, frequently is the first target. A purely fermentative order of digestion is disturbed by bacterial decomposition. Great amount of gas is produced, some of which comes into contact with the lungs by osmosis. Halitosis, or bad breath becomes noticeable.

The bacteria keep marching on. The gall bladder could provide ideal conditions for proliferation. The kidneys, bladder and sex organs are not exempt. In the female, the lower pelvis becomes a choice target for the germs to set up house.

The long chain of "itis" complaints are in the making.

What is the answer? To cut out the offending organ is certainly doing it the hard way. Also we cannot agree with Dr. Lane, who attacked the problem a little closer at the source by removing the colon—the birthplace of the bacteria.

Another way does exist. What is so remarkable, is that the other path is so simple, yet so demonstrably effective.

Having trained several thousand doctors in advanced healing methods over a period of twenty years, I feel I am somewhat qualified in making certain positive statements. In my approach to the doctors, I told them my training was free to them, if my teachings failed to bring improvements in their problem cases. Even a single disappointment establishing sufficient reason to forget about the fee.

The response of the doctors to the new orientation and treatment was overwhelming. Enlarged tonsils shrank like magic, with soreness abating. Chronic headaches disappeared, skin disorders cleared and "that tired feeling" was replaced by a bouyant feeling of well-being. Pituitary, thyroid or adrenal gland involvements also improved demonstrably as was observed in heart, liver, kidney and bladder. Better yet, the intestinal tract again assumed its normal functioning. Contrary to Lane's dictum, the colon had been permitted to exist, the new order afforded taming of the ambitious germs.

In mild cases of disorders, practically complete recoveries were inaugurated. In more advanced diseases, decided improvements in the condition could be realized. Yet, limitations in results of some cases had to be recognized. A famous German authority stated that if an organ is more than three-quarters destroyed, it could not regenerate.

This possibly explains the occasional flare-up of advanced chronic involvements when certain organs are far along the path of degeneration. But even in such serious cases, improvements can always be noted.

Balancing Metabolism

The question now becomes pertinent, just *what* is this system bringing about such remarkable changes? There are no hidden secrets involved, the principle of *balancing metabolism* always works.

Manipulations of bony and soft tissues help a great deal, especially in traumatic (injury) cases. Often one or two treatments may restore serious conditions of loss of equilibrium. Hip, neck or diverse joint troubles respond to speedy corrections. Pressure application (Neuropractic) as suggested in these pages will reward the user with relief of pain in a little time. often in a matter of minutes.

In chronic condition of any systemic disorder, manipulations alone are not enough to bring about lasting improvements. The entire mechanism of body chemistry must be overhauled from the ground up. Again how incredibly easy this can be accomplished. The "Royal treatment," *the fast,* always astounds both the patient and doctor with the result of speedy improvement. It is no wonder considering the colon—poison—bacteria relationship, and when you realize that the intestines become practically sterile in a matter of ten or so days under the fast.

Your New Diet Approach

When you resume eating, the new diet approach is followed. The emphasis now is directed to establish and maintain a state of friendly relationship between the busy colon workers and the rest of the body.

Let us shun all animal flesh, fish and eggs, and let us enjoy natural ripened fruit, seeds and vegetables, some sour milk and cheese with as little cooking as possible.

You still may and rightly are expected to be dubious. You reason that such a diet could be perfectly all right for the other fellow but that you yourself could not "sustain strength" on such a fare. Many hundreds of times I had to combat arguments along these lines, often to the point of frustration.

Then the thought struck me that no one wants to be told what to do. Let them make a short trial and then decide for themselves. I would point out that no one would starve by missing a few meals. They surely could fast for three or four days after which they could either quit or continue a little longer. A similar approach was used with the diet. There I became a little more insistent to request a trial period of two weeks.

Let result speak for itself. The human organism possesses such enormous recuperative powers that demonstrable improvements in body conditions definitely become apparent within the period of suggested trial time.

THE WHEAT BRAN COCKTAIL

In many impairments of the lungs, when there is coughing or difficulty of breathing, a definite lack of phosphorus has been detected. Healthy blood shows up to 9.5 percent of phosphorus in its total mineral content. This element is one of the key substances without which calcium cannot perform its functions.

If the phosphorus level in the body is low, the lungs will equally show a deficiency of the element. Normally, healthy lungs give an acid reaction with litmus paper, provided by phosphoric acid. In tuberculosis the lungs give a neutral or alkaline reaction due to the absence of phosphoric acid. In all cases of "TB" of the lungs a deposit of lime is found. This deposit sometimes becomes so great as to be called "chalky lungs." It would be impossible for the calcium to be deposited in the lung tissues, if the phosphorus level in the body had been maintained.

If we take an animal membrane, a bladder, and fill it with a solution of any mineral and hang it up, there will be no leakage through the skin; not a drop will appear on the outside of the bladder. We can let the solution remain in the bladder for days and it will guard its contents as safely as a glass bottle.

If we now take the filled bladder and immerse it in another solution of different density, the contents of the bladder will immediately begin to pass out through the walls of the bladder into the solution outside of the bladder. In the meantime the solution on the outside will pass through the bladder membrane into the inside, until both solutions are the same in character.

This process is called *osmosis*, it could also be called life. Osmosis is going on in the body at all times. It is the transfer of liquids through a membrane.

Every time we eat, we change the mineral make-up of the blood. In this way we keep changing the character of the fluid on the outside of the cells in order to keep it different from the fluid inside so that osmosis during life never ceases.

In mineral deficiencies, the fluids inside the cells and outside the cells become somewhat identical and osmosis becomes feeble. In mineral starvation, the fluids become entirely identical and death arrives.

Phosphorus, calcium, magnesium, iron, silica, etc. are plentifully supplied in Bran in an edible form. Not only lungs, but all bone structures, teeth, in fact the entire body desperately needs to maintain its structure by getting the minerals from a source where all the elements are presented in a balanced formula.

Bran Recipe

Remember Liebig's law that all components of nutrition must be present; that if even one single element is missing from the combination, nutrition can not serve its purpose. *Acquire the habit of stocking a generous supply of wheat bran. Take one cup of the bran and mix it in one quart of warm water. Let stand for 12 hours, strain and drink the liquid. Take this potion once daily for ten days and watch the resurgence of energy in your body.*

The bran is also used in connection with Kruska. Also, it can be sprinkled a little on salads, if some additional roughage is required in the intestinal tract to overcome sluggishness. Remember, the material may be too irritating to the lining of the bowels. In this case, do without the bran until the colitis has been overcome. Vegetable juices may then have to be used generously to help clear up the inflammation or irritation of the bowel.

6

The Use of Sea Water
for Health

Several years ago a brilliant agricultural engineer met a young mother devoting all of her time to her crippled son, age eleven. The boy was on crutches, could neither speak nor feed himself.

The engineer was keenly alerted to the problem of soil erosion and inexhaustible mineral supply in our seas. He suspected that there could be a relationship between deficient food and the poor condition of the child.

Perhaps seawater in small amounts could be added to the boy's diet, to see if such mineral supplementation would improve nutrition. The mother, receiving the seawater without cost, agreed to give the boy one ounce of it daily, with the food. By filtration the water had been treated in the removal of plankton and protozoa, etc.

The boy also had a little dog, equally sick, with mangey hair, watery eyes and "revolting halitosis." Both boy and dog received the water. After the second month, the boy showed improvement, he could walk a little without crutches, the dog also began to look much better. After four months, both boy and dog surprised everyone. The crutches now were discarded, the boy could walk without difficulty. The dog was full of vigor, with a shiny new coat.

A well known eye specialist made an experiment with seawater on his own body. The doctor was suffering from a cataract in his left eye. Nothing seemed to help the condition except surgical removal, which was contemplated in a short time.

The doctor had also been troubled with bursitis, a painful affliction in the shoulder joints.

In a period of nine months, not only the cataract disappeared, but also the shoulder condition, which had been suffered for twenty years.

Another well known physician used seawater on his family and patients. The doctor's elderly father had been a victim of Parkinson's disease for several years. He couldn't feed himself, even by spoon, because of his violent shakings.

The seawater was given. In two months, the old gentleman made such great improvements that he could feed himself and write letters.

What is the mysterious substance contained in seawater that brings about such startling improvements in diseases of man or beast?

In England, seawater was known as a remedy as early as the middle ages along the coasts. During the Eighteenth Century, when Russel founded the first sea bathing resort in Brighton, the water was used in drinking, as a poultice and in enemas.

The oceans are the world's greatest store house of minerals. So far, over sixty of the known elements have been discovered. In addition to these elements there exists another mysterious force in seawater, as yet not identified. It is a life-giving element that in some way may be associated with the chemo-electrical powers generated by the cosmic forces and transmitted to the oceans and the soil through the energies of the sun.

This life-giving substance loses its force through heat in a similar manner as that encountered with plants. It is the principle of creation, which up to now man has not mastered, and probably never will.

Seawater is a natural product and as such must be used. Cooking destroys the creative force in the water as in the egg. A cooked egg will not hatch.

Artificial seawater, made with strictest attempts to simulate the real thing, will not support life. Fish have been placed in large containers holding several hundred gallons of the man made water and the fish promptly died. In a subsequent experiment a little of real seawater was added—the fish then thrived.

Composition

Seawater, in an ionized form, is readily assimilated by the body. The composition is approximately the same as that of the liquids in the organism. It contains about three and one-half percent minerals of which table salt comprises seventy-eight percent, magnesium fifteen percent, calcium four percent and three percent all other minerals combined.

By the drinking of only one ounce of seawater daily, we are getting such infinitestimal, small amounts of the actual mineral substance, that it is not the crude minerals as such that bring on the good results. Some authorities think that it is the salts of the heavy metals with their catalytic actions which account for the health giving properties of seawater.

A Drastic Use of Sea Water

In my own experience in the use of seawater, I found similar gratifying results. A frantic phone request was received one day at the office, could a house call be made to attend to an elderly lady gravely ill? The patient was found to be in a most pitiful condition. Although of small stature, the lady was but a shadow of herself, weighing a little over sixty-five pounds from a normal weight of above one-hundred pounds.

It was a clear state of starvation, caused by her inability to digest food.

The patient complained that any kind of food, after ingestion, would create gas discomforts in such violent proportions as to be unable to be endured.

I was told that a private sanitarium had refused to admit the patient on the grounds that she was "too far gone." The examination did not reveal the presence of any lumps or masses in abdominal region. A puzzling case indeed.

A manipulative treatment was given. The patient was so weak, that she had to be helped, turning in bed. I had very little hope that she would survive the following day. Suddenly, seawater flashed into my mind, as a last resort it should be tried by all means.

A couple of days later the patient's husband phoned again and exuberantly told me that the treatment "had worked." For the first time in several weeks the suggested diet had been accepted without trouble and—enjoyed. From then on the frail little lady improved from day to day. In less than three months she regained her full strength and normal body weight.

My treatment undoubtedly contributed to the amazing turn-about in the condition of the emaciated patient. But I am firmly convinced that the use of seawater was the deciding factor in bringing about the speedy recovery.

Seawater Therapy for a Semi-Starved Patient

I am reminded of another case with certain similarities. A man called at the office, complaining also of not being able to take any kind of food without creating excruciating pains from gas disturbances. As a consequence, nutrition was practically at a standstill, the patient being in a semi-starved condition. Once of powerful build, with enormous chest development, he presented a grotesque picture when attempting to lie face down on the treatment table. Several pillows had to be used to prop up the abdomen to permit some support and take the weight away from the rib cage.

The man was told about the favorable results obtained from seawater in the case of the tiny little lady. A similar course of diet plus seawater was promptly adopted. Again, the results were surprising. The gas forming tendencies lessened as diges-tion and assimilation improved. The "hollowness" below his chest filled out and soon pillows were no longer required for support when lying on his stomach. The amounts of seawater taken were small. Three teaspoons—three times daily added to drinking water.

Again we must wonder about the exceedingly small doses of

the water, constituting an insignificant amount of minerals. Surely, the addition of these elements to the diet as such alone could not be the only reason for the speedy improvements observed.

The Secret of Sea Water

There remains no alternative than to realize that other principles are involved, as formerly mentioned. Could it be that the seawater made it possible to close the circuit of an electropotential arc? Could it be that the newly provided minerals acted as a switch for the body generating mechanism to establish contact with the *cosmic force?*

The behavior of nerve tissue, or for that matter the behavior of all body cells certainly point strongly in that direction.

The European medical doctors, practicing as homeopaths, appear to agree to such an orientation. Their adherence to prescribing infinitesimal small amounts of mineral or botanical substances correlates such an assumption. In some instances, the healing agents may be diluted as much as several thousand times. And yet, there are recorded many cases of amazing improvements.

The mineral components contained in seawater act as catalysts to re-organize disturbed body functioning. The secret of life creation is imparted in it and must be regarded as "living" matter such as is found in live plants or fertile eggs. Any temperature, high enough to create pain in our skin, will reduce the living force of seawater and eventually destroy it.

The use of seawater in burns is highly recommended. Any external sores or carbuncles will quickly respond with compresses saturated with the water.

Bleeding gums indicate a lack of mineral balance. The taking of seawater by mouth as well as massaging gums with the fluid will help.

Hemorrhoids or any other rectal difficulty have been treated with seawater enemas. After bowel cleansing, one half cup of it retained has brought lasting improvements.

Seawater can be obtained from health stores. If concentrated, see that process was carried out by vacuum—without the use of heat.

SEA VEGETATION

In this connection, seaweeds in the form of kelp or dulse should be considered, the former coming from the Pacific, the latter from the Atlantic ocean. I have found the Dulse variety, coming from Nova Scotia, as being more efficient, especially so if consumed in a powder state, one-half teaspoon per day. The taking of this substance could substitute for the seawater or vice versa.

7

What You Should Know About Meat in Your Diet

There is no question that animal flesh products do provide important nutritional substances. In cold climates of Northern countries meat served the purpose of survival of the races.

But there are so many "buts" that we should try to get along with as little flesh food as possible. The top figures of European nutrition flatly state that the intake of meat more than twice weekly is derogatory to the body, as well as speeding up the process of aging.

The meatless diet of the Seventh Day Adventists may be one of the reasons why, as a group, they suffer *forty percent fewer heart or vessel diseases* than the rest of the population. Another menace of meat are parasites and hormone drugs. It is asserted that at least one out of six persons throughout America is afflicted with trichinosis, caused by parasites. Five percent of those having the infection, die. The controversial sex hormone, diethyl stilbestrol, even though banned in many countries still is being used to raise chickens and beef cattle in this country.

THE SALTPETER DANGER

Since the flesh of the killed animal undergoes rapid changes of decay, many chemicals are used to slow it down. The use of saltpeter reduces the growth of bacteria. Its use, in connection with other chemicals, presents a serious health complication.

In this connection, we are reminded that saltpeter is often an ingredient of foods served in jails or other penal institutes. This supplement frequently is found necessary to control the sex urge of the inmates. It is an established fact that often-repeated suppressions bring on lasting effects.

The normal color of flesh coming from a dead animal is yellow grey, of little cosmetic appeal. The saltpeter camouflages this unsightly look with a lively pink or red.

While some of us may not be concerned about inclinations to sex proclivities, we must be reminded that the sex potential is the spark plug to the entire chain of the endocrine grands. Furthermore, damaging effects of substances contained in our foods do not necessarily confine themselves to attacking singular targets.

Besides saltpeter, there are other chemicals used as preservatives in meat. This in particular is the case in sausages. The term "embalmed" can rightly be applied.

I was told by one of my patients that at one time this lady had purchased several pounds of "frankfurters." The package had been misplaced and was found several weeks later on some forgotten shelf. Surprisingly, the thin, long sausages still looked invitingly red and were apparently free of decay. The lady's husband, a chemist, examined the heavily treated meat substances and became so shocked about the amount of chemical additives, that he whole-heartedly adopted the meatless diet.

SMOKED MEATS

Hams and other smoked meats, before smoking, are subjected to pickling. Again, saltpeter is one of the ingredients of the brine, plus a large amount of sugar, as well as borax and other chemicals.

In the incomplete combustion of wood in the smoke production, gases are developed belonging to the tar family. Here we find carbolic acid, creosote, formaldehyde, etc. which partially penetrate the meat. These tar derivatives are in no way removed from the meat after the completion of the smoking process and therefore become a part of the food.

This might be dangerous for some people, like smoking tobacco.

While dictating these lines, a thought flash suddenly entered my mind. For several years I had known a vivacious young lady, full of fun, a fine housekeeper and devoted wife of a friend. The woman was well-educated, a witty conversationalist, a boon to any party.

The lady agreed with most of my theories in nutrition except that of eating meat. She was particularly partial to smoked hams with their "delicate taste and nut like flavor."

There were three in the family, husband, wife and one child. a good sized ham was usually purchased every week, to be consumed in several stages the following days.

Then the sad event happened to the lady. I had been away on a regular teaching itinerary. All of a sudden the lady had become ill suffering from extreme bloatings in abdomen. The old story: quick rush to the hospital, x-ray treatments and—death. The husband was so grieved by the loss of his wife, that he also followed her into the grave in a short time.

On my return, one of our mutual acquaintances told me the tragic story. On her deathbed, my steadfast antagonist finally saw the light and told the party that she knew then the real cause of her plight. If I had only listened to the "good doctor" was her often heard remark.

We must also consider a high speed process, in which the smoking is finished in thirty-six to forty-eight hours. Instead of smoke, a brownish liquid is used made out of wood vinegar, creosote and other tar substances dissolved in water. The previously pickled meat is placed in this fluid and is ready to be sold within less than two days.

In my practice, many times I had occasion to watch results of curtailing the meat intake to better body conditions.

Kidney and bladder cases invariably show the speediest improvement. This "having to get up at night" business always responds by fewer trips to the bathroom. In many cases, the patients could sleep through the entire night without interruptions.

Still the biggest implication in meat consumption is the disposition of the colon bacteria. Each morsel of meat will help to set off another colony of the putrefactive type. With the diet reform, it is possible that the decay principle can be sufficiently controlled especially if other adequate nutritional caution is employed at the same time.

At any rate, I am convinced that man not only can live *with-*

out eating animal flesh but can do so much better to the benefit of increased well-being.

My patients have proven this, as well as observations in my own use and that of my family.

A CONVINCING EXPERIMENT

At the University hospital in Tuebingen, Germany, Professor Mueller has introduced a research method of microscopic examination of the capillaries, those fine thread blood vessels. Even with a magnification of only sixty, the eye sees in the skin through the horny layer the fine hairpin-like loops of the smallest blood vessels which exist in the human body. These capillaries are the trade ports and trans-shipping stations of the tissues and organs for the receiving of nourishment and disposal of waste products.

Through the microscope the eye also sees the streaming blood and is able to observe the speed of its flow.

A nutritional experiment was made on two young students. First their "capillary pictures" were recorded, they looked normal. Each of them was given then over a period of ten days a daily diet of three pounds of meat of all kinds and wide variety, together with one ounce of white bread and lemonade.

At the end of ten days their capillary pictures were again recorded.

Result: The capillaries had swollen into broad elongated bags, ruptured in places by blood diffusing out into the surrounding tissue. The blood stream was slowed down and the blood itself congested.

A scorbutic swelling of the gums in the mouth had set it, so that they bled easily. A similar condition of the capillaries was found in all other parts of the body.

It took a meatless diet of over one month's duration to bring about a gradual return of the vessels to their normal condition!

Thus in a short period of only ten days, a one-sided meat diet had appreciably damaged most vital structures of *youthful* bodies. What a one-sided meat diet manages to do in ten days, regular meat diets will accomplish in twenty or thirty years.

8

The Smoking
Problem

John Wayne, the famous movie actor, recently created a big sensation when he suddenly emerged from a hospital, apparently cured from a lung cancer. Contrary to the wishes of the studio's publicity department, which attempted to hush up the matter, America's he-man image insisted on "telling it all."

John Wayne reportedly had smoked five packs of cigarettes a day, a generous amount, even for a chain smoker. The inevitable consequences, chronic irritation and cancer. A lengthy hospital stay plus surgical removal of the cancerous portion of the lung followed.

With characteristic frankness, the actor told the world about his "toughest fight" in all of his life. He said he "licked it" and projected the warning for others to keep from making the same mistake.

Emerson Foote resigned a top position with a large advertising agency, in protest against cigarette promotion. His reason: he did not want to encourage people to "kill themselves." Mr. Foote said that the advertising budget amounted to two-hundred million dollars a year. He reportedly asserted that cigarette smoking kills up to 300,000 people a year.

Tobacco and its smoke contains over twenty-eight poisons. Doctors and laboratory experts have analyzed and denounced it as a narcotic more dangerous than morphine. Responsible physicians in Europe have proclaimed the tobacco habit as the "brown pest." It affects all body cells, particularly of the brain, poisons the blood stream, and furnishes an environment

153

for disease, accidents, crimes, delinquency and similar conditions leading to degeneration.

Over two-thirds of our population has been reduced to a
state of tobacco addiction by high pressure advertising. The
cash outlay is Four Billion dollars per year!

It is not only men or boys that smoke, over forty percent of
our girls and women also have adopted the habit. The powerful effect of television, with its hypnotic spell to conformity,
has taken its mark.

Only a few decades ago smoking was abhored by women.
But the tricky slogans of the clever hucksters did the trick.
Slogans projected "harmless pleasures, keeping slender, relaxed
and fashionable." It was suggested that smoking made women
more alluring to men which made so many of the fairer sex
fall into the trap.

It is difficult for man to free himself from the grip of tobacco
addiction. It is much more difficult for a woman to do so
because she possesses a more highly organized nervous system. In a similar proportion the damage in her case is more
far-reaching in the harmful effects to her nerves and general
undermining of her health.

What is this mysterious "lift" and imagined "pleasure" sup-
posedly experienced by the smoker? Decidedly they are
imaginations or illusions of the disturbed mind caused by the
drug and poisons. The first effect of smoking is confusion. The
smoker doesn't know one way or the other whether he feels
pleasure or pain, whether he is being lifted up or let down, or
stimulated or relaxed.

One of the greatest misapprehensions about smoking is that
it is a stimulant—in fact it is a severe depressant.

The apparent lift the smoker feels is in reality a letdown
with the constant demand on body reserves needed to counteract the intake of poisons. The adrenal glands play an important
part in this drama of maintaining the forces of life. This gland
pours adrenalin into the blood stream in order for the liver to
respond and release the stored-up sugar into the blood. This
is a kind of borrowing which never pays back because the
effects of smoking do not add anything in the way of nourishment, to give the deceptive lift. It is true that nicotine for a

short time does increase the blood sugar level. But so does strychnine, for that matter!

Tobacco addiction is so severe that some patients continue to smoke even though they suffer agonizing pain from gangrene of arms or legs. In one case one patient lost all four extremities because he would not give up smoking. Such a condition is commonly known as Buerger's disease, also termed the smoker's disease. The poisons in tobacco degenerate cells and vessels of the feet or hands, creating a condition known as gangrene. The disease starts often with the soreness of toes which the smoker usually passes off as a touch of athlete's foot. The flesh continues to decompose in the feet, and the gangrene spreads through the rest of the body relentlessly.

We have mentioned that there are twenty-eight poisons in tobacco. Taking but a single one, nicotine, an experiment demonstrated the immense destructive power of this drug. A smoker takes about three milligrams of nicotine into his body every time he smokes an average cigarette. This amount is enough to kill a man instantly if taken at once.

The reason that this killing action is not instantaneous, is because much of the smoke escapes into the air where others have to breathe it. When a cigarette is smoked, thirty-five percent of nicotine is lost in the side stream of smoke. Twenty-two percent enters the mouth through the main stream of the smoke, the remainder is in the unsmoked portion of the cigarette. Of the twenty-two percent which enters the mouth, not all of it reaches the breathing passages. When smoke is held in the mouth for two seconds, up to three-quarters of it is absorbed. When the smoke is inhaled, up to ninety-six percent of the nicotine is absorbed.

These figures should present a potent argument against those who profess to receive little damage from the smoking since they do not inhale. Read the figures above again.

The filter promotion has done much to lull the unsuspecting public into a false sense of security. Filter tips have been investigated and denounced as frauds, making believe that the tars and nicotine are filtered out entirely or at least below the danger margin.

In a national survey it was pointed out that tar reductions

ranging from seven to seventeen percent are too small to be really significant in terms of health protection. Even if the filter did remove all the nicotine, there are still a number of other poisons left in the smoke which can not be filtered. To name but one is arsenic, with which the tobacco plants are liberally sprayed as deadly insecticides. The public health service stated that these poison sprays are not removed from the plants.

In a test made on various brands of cigarettes on the market, it was found that the arsenic content of five leading brands was practically the same. Arsenic dehydrates the blood, lungs, liver, kidneys and destroys nerve sensitivity. A dried-up nervous system brings on premature old age.

A seven percent solution of arsenic poison is also found in the cigarette paper according to research chemists.

The effects of smoking on motherhood is devastating. Nicotine is excreted in the milk of nursing mothers. Smoking women had more painful menstruation and earlier change of life with more complications than non-smokers. Even women who did not smoke but handled tobacco were poisoned to some extent, had difficulties with their pelvic organs, and irregularities at childbirth. For example, in a tobacco factory of Brazil, women had a higher rate of miscarriage, stillbirths, and vomiting than women outside the factory.

9

The County
Without a Toothache

A few years ago there appeared several articles in national magazines about a town and county where there was much less tooth trouble than in any other part of America. Dental cavities were practically unknown, even in old age people having enviable sets of all their teeth without any signs of decay.

The term fluorine was often mentioned, as this element had been demonstrated to exist in generous amounts throughout the area.

The ensuing intense publicity immediately connected the extraordinary tooth health with the fluorine contents of the soil, which inaugurated the controversial fluoridation program throughout the Westernized World.

Deafsmith County lies at an altitude of 4,000 feet. The soil consists of "blow soils" several feet thick, which had been blown in during the past several hundred thousand years.

Below this accumulated top soil we find large beds of limestone with interspaced shale formations. All of this indicates the presence of an ancient marine bed which, over a period of millions of years, has been pushed up to the present level.

One of my students, a retired dentist, made some investigations on soil compositions and found that the particular region had been heavily enriched with kelp beds.

Here again, we find the chain reaction of cosmic forces being "preserved" for later use. Through the sun and photosynthesis, every element contained in seawater is stored in a concentrated ionized form. With the uplift of the land, the sea vegetation

157

becomes a part of the soil, explaining the unusual fertility of the land.

The presence of calcium fluoride is only one of the about sixty elements so far identified in the soil. In addition, there is calcium, potassium, magnesium, in fact every substance existing in the oceans, and for that matter known to exist in the universe.

What makes the Deafsmith soils so ideal for the growing of health promoting foods is the presence of all needed mineral components plus their exact balance in proportions to each other.

Another contributing factor is the elevation, climate and sun. There is an abundance of brilliant sunshine which strikes the plants with greater intensity than in the lower altitude, due to lower humidity.

The water in Deafsmith County is said to be the finest in the country. The mineral enrichment again is demonstrable.

The percentage of men accepted by the Army in Deafsmith County is possibly the highest in America. In June, 1944, ninety-three percent of those called had passed the physical examination, compared to less than fifty percent of the National average. The high percentage also included those who had migrated to the county from other areas.

The foods grown in Deafsmith County are of highest quality, finest taste and produced in abundant amounts. Most nutritious carrots have been raised, yielding seventeen tons per acre. Wheat or other grains show a much higher protein content than those grown in other regions.

FLUORIDATION

We have learned about calcium fluoride being one of the components found in the waters of Deafsmith County. The implications of perfect tooth structures became an enticing subject to be projected into other areas.

The aluminum industry with its huge waste stockpile of sodium fluoride, quickly saw the opportunity and went into action. That their product was entirely different from the natural substance did not seem to concern them. It is a highly virulent toxin used as rat poison. When added to water, making hydrofluoric acid, it is used for etching glass. Sodium fluoride is an inorganic poison eighty-five times more toxic than calcium fluoride, of organic origin.

The inorganic waste product in the production of aluminum is most difficult to handle, because of its corrosiveness. As rat killer and insecticide it was sold for one and one-half cents per pound.

Now appeared the prospect of dumping the dangerous by-product into the water supply of the nation. Not only would this solve the disposition of the corrosive substance, it would equally permit the increase of revenue ten times the former amount.

Sodium fluoride is a compound of sodium and fluorine. Sodium is a metal and very unstable. Fluoride is one of the halogens. It is a gas, one of the most untameable of all the elements. It attacks most anything and combines with more elements than any other known element. When the two elements combine to form sodium fluoride, the compound constitutes one of the most deadly poisons known to man.

When taken into the human system as in drinking water, not all of it is excreted. A part of it is retained and accumulated in the tissues like arsenic or lead is retained.

Sodium fluoride has the property of settling out calcium. The incidence of arthritis is increased because some of the calcium is deposited in the joints and cartilages. The substance impairs the functions of the pancreas, liver and kidneys. All enzyme activities in the body are damaged by it and even the enamel of the teeth is attacked in the process.

FLUORIDATION ECONOMICS

The proponents for fluoridation admit that it will help only the teeth of children of twelve and under, and only partially. It is difficult to see why the entire water system of a city is to be engaged to carry the "helping substance" to a small fraction of one percent of all users of the water. In the event the medication *did* work would it not be more practical to dispense the material or the treated water separately to those who could benefit by it? In this connection, Mr. Rodale, the famous health authority remarked so pointedly: "It is like shipping a single pill to a patient with a twenty ton truck." A similar evaluation was voiced by a first class water engineer who was appalled by the unrealistic economy of the fluorine distributing method. "What would you think of a doctor who told you to buy six-hundred bottles of medicine, use one of the bottles and pour the other five-hundred and ninety-nine bottles down the drain?"

The whole fluoridation controversy has been succinctly expressed by a former president of the American Dental Association in Oral Hygiene. "The main causes of tooth decay, as every dentist knows, are candy, soft drinks and refined foods. Why not prohibit, by suitable laws, the manufacture of refined sugar, refined flour, and similar devitalized atrocities?"

10

Cholesterol and Lecithin

Among our average middle-aged American males, one out of five develops a heart attack. A few of those completely recover, but others remain what are known as "cardiac cripples." They have to slow down to a restricted pattern of life for the rest of their lives. People who are overweight suffer twice as many heart involvements as people with normal weight.

What Is Cholesterol?

Cholesterol which is found in all animal tissues, is one of the chief causes of heart disease. It is a substance resembling chewing gum and builds up within the inside walls of blood or lymph vessels. The resulting narrowing of space in the vessels favors the formation of blood clots, cutting off the supply line to a part of the heart and brings on the attack. Should the blocked vessels belong to the brain, the results will be stroke.

Lecithin Controls Cholesterol

The presence of cholesterol in the body is essential to all body functions. It is not the normal amount we are concerned with, but its excess. A perfectly operating control mechanism keeps the cholesterol amounts to ideal levels under all conditions and times. The control substance is *Lecithin*. This material is found in grains, beans, natural fats and egg yolks. Both cholesterol and lecithin are contained in eggs, animal fats in

161

their natural state and vegetable oils that have not been chemically treated.

In the cooking process of prepared food, the heat does not affect the cholesterol, but destroys the lecithin. Natural butter contains both cholesterol and lecithin. But in the process of pasteurizing, lecithin is destroyed, leaving only cholesterol. A similar situation is repeated in all foods containing both substances, when the controlling factor is killed by the heat. A good example is furnished by animal flesh. Cats fed exclusively on cooked meat will sicken and die in a short time. Post-mortem examination reveals destructive changes in blood vessels known as artherosclerosis. On a diet of raw meat, the animals will thrive. This explains the high incidence of heart or vessel involvements of meat eaters, who would not think of eating the meat in a raw state. The Eskimos, consuming their flesh foods uncooked, are unaware of cholesterol infusion or vessel damage, even though displaying a much shorter life span than other races, subsiding on less meat in-take in their diets.

Cholesterol teaches man a potent lesson in dietetics. Since it is unthinkable to eat meat in the raw state, and since the heating process destroys the disease preventing components, animal flesh is not well suited for human consumption.

The cholesterol implication becomes still more involved when connecting it to the fat or oil consumption.

The Hydrogenation Process in Commercial Foods

About fifty years ago, a French chemist received the Nobel Prize for his discovery of rendering fat substances free of rancidity or organic decay. The process originally had been intended for use in soap manufacture. Ship loads of coconut oils from tropical countries often arrived in various states of composition.

The chemist devised a method whereby the oily substance is placed in boilers, subjected to high pressure, hydrogen and heat. With the use of powdered nickel as a catalyst or "hastener," the once unsightly and smelly mass is attacked. When removed from the boiler, the material has the appearance of axle grease, a dark colored, gooey mess. It is then bleached with corrosive chemicals to finish the change from an organic to an inorganic substance; from a live to a dead concoction. Oils coming from nuts and seeds that may have decayed during periods of transportation, are processed to again take their place in nutrition for humans. That the new product not only turned into a synthetic commodity, but could consitute a *health peril* was of little concern to anyone.

It was found that slaughter houses could equally benefit from the new treatment. Left-overs of fat receive the cosmetic improvement by the application of hydrogen processing.

Now, oil and fat assumed a glistening white appearance. Storage problems such as rancidities or other organic changes had been completely overcome. The treatment was called *hydrogenation* and revolutionized the food processing industry. Originally intended to be used by the soap makers, the process was found to have been made to order for canners, or packers of foods. It was learned that hydrogenated fats could be put into a container where it could remain on the grocer's shelf for months, years—or forever. Furthermore, the refined substance exerted a strange preserving effect on other processed "foods" with which it was blended.

This explains the wide use of hydrogenated fats. It is contained in most bakery goods, potato chips, peanut butter and practically all processed foods.

What is the answer? *Shun* all processed foods. Use sunflower seeds, sesame seeds, flaxseeds and other seeds that have not been chemically treated. Get whole walnuts, hazelnuts, brazil nuts, pine nuts, almonds, etc. and shell them as needed immediately *before* consuming them. Obtain whole kernels of grain and permit the outside hulls to act as protectors to the contained inner food. All nuts and grains are seeds and as such are endowed with life giving properties. They were intended by nature to provide perfect nutrition for man, in connection with green leaves, stems, tubers and roots. Certainly not by hydrogenation!

No special mention is made of fruits, because they are essentially seeds. The delectable outside soft or meaty portion constitutes the energy providing components so perfectly balanced to the seeds in its attractive form.

For salad oils, insist on obtaining cold pressed, natural varieties such as saf-flower, sesame, sunflower, olive, etc.

In the event of possible existing cholesterol infusions, lecithin, as a food supplement, brings about certain effects of detergent action on cholesterol.

In animal experimentations, injections of lecithin resulted in the removal of cholesterol deposits in arteries.

11

The Wonderful World of
Corrective Foods and Herbs

There were a number of times in my practice when truly baffling cases presented themselves. Often, serious nerve afflictions had been noted in patients living under normal conditions, abstaining from coffee, tea, drugs or animal flesh foods. Most of the patients were from farms where regular poisonous sprays had been used to treat the soil and crops several times per year.

In one case, a bleeding "ulcer" in chest always became more acute after spraying. In another case both man and wife were nearly paralyzed after each "dusting" by plane. In following my advice, both parties sold or leased their places and moved into uncontaminated areas, with a corresponding speedy correction of their condition.

I recently received a notice from Ecuador, South America. Millions of fish in coastal rivers died, creating a catastrophical dilemma for the native Indians subsisting from the fish.

Jungle forests had been destroyed to make room for the banana trees, without regard to maintaining plant coverings of the soil. The usual heavy rains, no longer permitted to soak into the ground, ran off. The more disastrous effect followed. Heavy doses of Toxaphene and other pesticides had been used and washed into the rivers. The acquatic life congregation came to an abrupt end.

The organic approach to the raising of crops is the answer. Soil management through mulching and compost will raise crops' resistance to pests. If necessary, botanical and harmless agents can control the few "bugs" that could be present on crops produced in healthy soils.

HERBS AND FRUITS

In my discussion about aches and pains and their removal from the body, certain botanicals should be included, having demonstrable healing qualities.

We shall become acquainted with one member of this category, Comfrey, which I believe possesses hightest attributes regarding our good health.

The Uses of Comfrey

I am referring to comfrey, which can be grown most everywhere, having originated in the Caucasus mountains in Southern Russia.

Comfrey is a plant, the leaves and roots having been used for centuries to alleviate pains, reduce congestion and heal open sores. An old English directory describes in glowing terms this herb as containing the property of "glueing together" wounds.

Back in the Seventeenth Century a bone-setter became famous by treating fractures with a pulp made of the scraped root spread upon old muslin which was wrapped around the limb and bandaged over. It soon stiffened, supporting and strengthening the part. The bandage was not removed until the limb became well.

The *British Medical Journal* of June 8, 1912 reported the amazing recovery of a "hopeless" case of a man, age 83. The patient had advanced hardening of arteries, low temperature, with blood in the urine. An ulcer appeared on the left foot, spreading rapidly until large parts of bones became exposed. The patient became delirious and was removed to his home to die.

He was then treated with several fomentations, saturated with a decoction made out of comfrey root. The ulcer promptly began to heal, with the patient making corresponding improvements.

Dr. Murray, of the Liverpool hospital confirmed the astounding values of comfrey in the treatment of large numbers of men who had been badly burned in an explosion at a factory.

The burns were mostly of the second and third degree.

Comfrey was tried first on only two cases. Results were so outstanding that the herb treatment was adopted for all other cases with greatest success.

The plant contains a specific healing agent, known as Allantoin, present in both roots and leaves. This substance has the ability as a cell—proliferent, making the edges of wounds grow together and healing sores.

Taken as a tea, it helps to overcome gastric or duodenal ulcers, or any irritation affecting small or large intestine.

The decoction for a supply is made by steeping one ounce of crushed comfrey root in one quart of water. The herb is also taken in a powder form, in cases of sore throats, hoarseness, etc. Internally, comfrey is introduced as a tea, concentration being equal in other herbal teas.

Comfrey embraces still another valuable attribute. That is besides its healing properties, the herb can be used as a most delectable green salad leaf. Its nutritional qualifications are most impressive, in comparison to alfalfa it contains nearly twice as much protein, about fifty percent higher mineral content and is decidedly rich in carotene, the forerunner of Vitamin A. It can also make a very good vegetable, prepared similarly to spinach.

Its roots go down ten feet tapping water during drought and gathering nutrients. It is easily raised and has no known insect pests.

Its technical name is Symphytum Peregrinum and it is strongly suggested that all of us should raise this health provoking plant in our garden, backyard or wherever a piece of ground is available.

In ancient Greece the physicians used herbs and fruits in treating disease. There are many amazing properties contained in our humble plants and ordinary trees all adopted to adjust the workings of the body when used with common sense.

In contrast we find the synthetic remedies, which, while suppressing the symptoms of the disorder, do not remove the cause of the disease. Often vital organs are damaged as exemplified in remedies for sleeplessness and their harmful effect on the nervous system.

THE APPLE

This king of the fruits has come into the limelight of medical explorations.

Dysentery is a severe intestinal affliction, often terminating fatally. In a case of acute intestinal catarrh, a patient had been suffering for over one month; he was emaciated and exhausted. The hospital physician had heard of a man who had cured himself very quickly of a similar severe condition by a diet of grated raw apple. It was decided to try the "apple cure." Astoundingly, within two days the patient recovered.

Many European hospitals are using the apple diet in most upsets of the digestive tract.

In my own experiences I have observed many cases, paralleling those mentioned above. About three pounds of apples are consumed daily, *with peels and seeds.* Nothing else taken, except water, if desired.

Apples contain great amounts of volatile substances—fruit acids, minerals, tannic acid, pectin, etc. The latter substance causes blood to congeal. This property alone may explain the speedy improvement in cases of mucous membrane involvement (dysentery). The apples act as a sponge in the intestine, absorbing toxic material for quick removal. In the meantime, the healing process goes on.

The apples are *grated* and immediately consumed in a *raw* state. Even when slightly cooked, the apple seems to exert healing action. In one resort, doctors had good results in the treatment of metabolic disorders, heart and vessel disease and dropsy. The patients received three pounds of stewed apples daily, with a little honey, three times per day, three days in each week.

JUNIPER BERRIES

The juniper berry is an ancient remedy for many ailments. The active principle of the berry is a volatile oil which dilates the capillaries of the mucous membranes of the digestive tract. As a result, the blood flow to the involved organs is increased with corresponding improvement to general metabolism. The volatile oils are fatal to bacteria and since soluble in fats, penetrate into bodies of bacteria.

The following is the juniper "cure" as used in a famous European resort. On first day, five berries are taken, on second day six, the third seven and so on until fifteen berries are taken daily. From then on one berry is taken less per day until down to five again. The berries are chewed three times per day. It is asserted that this treatment purifies the most unhealthy blood stream if repeated a few times.

To Relieve Arthritic Pains

One pound of juniper berries is soaked in six quarts of hot water. Next morning, boil for thirty minutes. Strain and use liquid for compresses, applied to painful areas as hot as can be borne.

WILLOW BARK

In World War II there was a shortage of drugs in Germany. It was known that Willow Bark contains the substance *salicin* which the body converts into *salicylic acid* to alleviate pain.

In a widely conducted experiment, willow bark was used in the treatment of arthritis and rheumatism, both acute and chronic with over seventy percent of cases reported as healings.

The synthetic preparation, *Aspirin,* on the other hand is not as beneficial to mucous membranes and capillaries. In addition, it has other certain side effects on the human organism as verified in any medical book on toxicology.

Willow bark is taken by steeping ½ ounce of it in three cups of boiling water. Allow to stand overnight, then boil for five minutes. Drink during day.

The bark can also be powdered in which case the tea need not be boiled. Take two teaspoons of powdered bark in three cups of boiling water. Let stand for eight hours and take after meals.

In some cases, willow bark can be mixed in equal amounts with birch leaves, prepared in a similar way and taken three cups during course of day.

The German medical experiment with willow bark demonstrated the overwhelming superiority of a natural healing agent to its synthetic counterpart, aspirin. One is speedily effective, alleviating pain and affording healing *without* afflicting harm to the organism—the other providing *temporary paralysis* to nerve tissues, *blocking* sensations of pain. One is constructive, the other destructive as admitted by top authorities. Remember, only God can make a tree, the chemist can make an artificial egg, but he cannot make it hatch.

THE OAK

Known as the sacred tree in ancient times, the active ingredient in oak is *tannin* which has astringent qualities. In cases of bronchial catarrh, diarrhea and hemorrhoids it is used as follows: one-half ounce of powdered oak boiled for ten minutes in one pint of water. A little honey may be added for sweetening.

For bladder condition take ⅓ ounce powdered bark and one teaspoon of crushed juniper berries boiled for five minutes in one-half pint of water. Three tablespoons are taken morning and evening with a little honey.

For external purposes take one ounce of powdered bark boiled in three pints of water for thirty minutes (two pints will remain). This solution can be used as a gargle for sore throat and swollen tonsils and as a fomentation for boils or skin eruptions. It is also useful for the feet with unpleasant odor.

A douche for personal hygiene for women, it can be used by boiling one part of oak bark in fifteen parts of water for thirty minutes.

THE BIRCH

This beautiful tree contains many healing properties in its leaves. The active ingredient is a diuretic. The famous professor Winternitz has shown that the *quantity of urine is often increased by eight times.* This extra functioning of the kidneys is not accomplished by the slightest irritation. It was also demonstrated that the excretion of albumin in the urine was lessened.

Dr. Jaennicke used the tea for *kidney stones* with great success. He found that the general condition of the patient was greatly improved after a period of treatment and that the *stones were passed* at first in pieces the size of a pea and later sand.

The tea is made with one teaspoonful of dried, finely cut birch leaves to each cup of water. Infuse in boiling water. The tea is taken on an empty stomach, one cup in the morning, one cup in the afternoon.

Professor Bohn used the tea for rheumatism, gout and kidney disease. He claims that the active agent in the tea *dissolves uric acid.* This substance called *sabonin,* is rich in potassium salts, which account for the diaphoretic results achieved.

THE ELDER

The tree came from Central Europe and was regarded sacred. Before the coming of Christianity, everyone passing the elder bush had to salute either by taking off the hat or bowing the head as a token of reverence. The people had discovered that in the elder they could find a cure for many ills.

The root supplies a laxative, the bark soothes inflammations, the leaves are used for burns and the berries are employed as a diuretic. The active ingredient of the elder is a volatile oil which encourages perspiration. Also contained is a *sex hormone* said to be beneficial in the climacteric. In addition, the berries are rich in Vitamin C.

The tea is made by taking two tablespoons of the flowers and infuse in one pint of water. Let stand for twenty minutes and "enjoy" with a little honey and lemon juice.

CAMOMILE (Anthemis Nobilis)

This is another medicinal plant with which we should become acquainted. The active ingredient is a volatile oil and glucoside having specific relaxing properties. Ever since the days of Disocorides, the Greek physician, camomile has been used to relieve the pains of *childbirth* and *menstruation*.

Dr. Steinmeltz has established that camomile tea can double the *flow of bile*. As a poultice or compress, the tea is beneficial in irritations of the skin such as eczema. For sleeplessness, a tea of equal portions of camomile, hops and salvia are brought to a boil.

HAWTHORN

The active ingredients in this shrub are tannin and saponin, besides a great number of rare trace elements. It has been scientifically established that the flower and fruit are a nonpoisonous remedy for heart or blood vessel conditions. Some doctors in Europe claim that hawthorn tea is *superior to digitalis* for "heart" patients.

One tablespoon of equal amounts of the flower and the fruit to one cup water. Drink during day in small doses.

YARROW (Achillea Mille Folium)

The active ingredient of yarrow is a substance helpful in menstrual difficulty, kidney and bladder trouble and said to *dissolve kidney stones*. The tea also has a toning up effect on skin. In England, it is used as a beauty preparation. It is claimed that washing the face in yarrow tea will allow the skin to become firm as well as prevent lines or wrinkles.

The tea is also used for control of bedwetting, chronic enlarged liver and bleeding hemorrhoids.

Take one tablespoon of the flowers plus two-thirds ounce of leaves to three cups of boiling water.

It is also stated that the tea is helpful for people who have sensations of numbness in hands and feet.

LADY'S MANTLE (Alchemilla Vulgaris)

This herb has been used for centuries as an excellent healer for sores and as a remedy for epilepsy.

It has also been employed to combat *excessive menstrual flow*.

Use five teaspoons of the cut up herb in one pint of water, boil it for two minuts. Drink two cups daily. If the herb is mixed with equal parts of cowslip, a very fine tea will result, excelling in aroma and flavor.

HEATHER

This is an ancient remedy for *cough* as well as general pain.

During the last war, pillows for wounded soldiers in Germany were filled with heather, inducing sound sleep in spite of pain.

Only the tips of the branches bearing the flowers are used, one-third ounce to one cup of water, boiled for two minutes.

DANDELION

Here we have not only an efficient healing agent, but equally a most nutritious food. The herb was used by the old physicians as an eye remedy. The Greek name for it (taraxacum) means "cures eye disease."

Dandelion is one of the richest sources of minerals with a high content of potassium and many trace elements. The specific ingredients are saponin and colocynthin which explain glandular improvements, particularly to liver and gall bladder with this herb.

For promoting increased urine and bile, take two tablespoons of dried leaves and roots boiled for five minutes in one pint of water. Take two cups daily.

As a food, fresh dandelion leaves are added to the daily salad.

COLTSFOOT (Tussilage Farfara)

This is another efficient remedy for *coughs and asthma.* For coughs, take one-quarter ounce of coltsfoot leaves infused in cup of boiling water. Let stand for ten minutes and strain.

For Asthma

Three parts of coltsfoot, three parts sage and three parts plantain. One-half ounce of this mixture infused in one pint of boiling water, strain after 15 minutes and sweeten with honey. One tablespoon is taken every hour.

THE STINGING NETTLE

In this humble plant we find even richer supplies of minerals than are contained in the dandelion. The plant is generously endowed with Vitamins A, C, and the B complexes. Nettle juice or nettle tea has been successfully employed to help rid the body of kidney or bladder stones. Best results have been obtained with nettle juice.

On account of the large amounts of chlorophyll and iron, the nettle can serve as a most nutritious spinach. Young nettles are washed and placed in a covered pan without water, using a little butter. In a few minutes the nettle will be ready and appreciated as a delectable dish.

Cold tea made from dried leaves is an excellent *beverage.* One-half ounce of leaves are infused in one quart of boiling water. Let stand for fifteen minutes and strain.

DECOCTION FOR STOMACH ULCERS

Take three pints of hot water and soak in it three-quarters cup of wheat bran and two-thirds cup of whole linseed overnight. In the morning boil for twenty minutes, until thick and slimy, from time to time thinning it down with a little water. Boil for 20 minutes in three pints of water one pound of unpeeled potatoes. Mix both concoctions while still hot and strain.

During first ten days of treatment, my stomach ulcer sufferers receive one cup of this mixture plus one-half cup of raw carrot juice every two hours, or 7 times during day.

ALKALINE DRINK FOR DIGESTIVE DISORDERS

Two pounds of various root vegetables, plus potatoes with peeling, carrots, celery, parsley, etc., are cleaned, cut up and boiled for 30 minutes in three quarts of water without salt. The liquid is strained to which is added two cups of wheat bran and one cup of whole linseed, allowed to stand overnight. On following morning, two cups of this mixture is taken, well-stirred to insure all the bran and linseed is swallowed with the drink.

LAXATIVE BREAKFAST OR LUNCH

One-quarter cup wheat bran, one-quarter cup whole linseed, one tablespoon ground barley, a few cut up figs, raisins and prunes are boiled in one cup of water for five minutes.

The dish is served with buttermilk or yogurt and honey to suit taste with stewed fruit or berries.

POTATO SENSATION

Large, well scrubbed potatoes are grated, skin and all, over a pan of boiling water. Boil until the porridge thickens and remove from heat. Most of the potatoes will be only half cooked, which is the purpose of this preparation.

Serve with sour milk, ground nuts and a green salad.

A GOOD SOURCE OF CALCIUM FOR YOUR DIET

Place two washed eggs in china bowl with the juice of four lemons. Put bowl in cool place and cover with a plate. Turn eggs every other day. After six days the lemon juice will have drawn the calcium out of the eggs, which can be discarded. Two tablespoons of the juice is taken every day. Every third day, two more eggs are placed and more lemon juice has to be added to keep the volume constant.

HOW TO MAKE AND USE SAUERKRAUT

Lactic acid is extremely important in providing a media for beneficial bacteria growth in the body, having a counteracting effect upon putrefaction in the colon. My objection to commercial sauerkraut is the heavy amounts of table salt used in its preparation. Following are two recipes overcoming the salt implications.

1. One bushel of white cabbage, one cup of juniper berries.

A small wooden barrel or large earthenware crock is required, also wooden lid, heavy weight (stone) and clean towel. Container and accessories must be sterilized with boiling water. Cabbage leaves are washed and cut into thin shreds. Place layer of three inches of cabbage on bottom of container and crush with stone *until juice runs out and a broth is formed.* Sprinkle a few juniper berries and put in the second layer, repeating the process until the container is nearly full. A few large cabbage leaves are put on top and covered with a clean towel.

On top of that put a few leaves with ventilation holes in them. Put the lid on and weight it down with the heavy stone used for crushing, which will press down the layers. It is important that all the layers be covered by the juice.

The container is placed in a warm room, in order for fermentation to start as quickly as possible. Cover the container with a clean sheet to protect it from dust. After a few days, and then every two or three days, remove all the scum. Each time, wash the cloth, the lid and the stone in boiling water. When the scum no longer rises, the process of fermentation is finished and the container can be put in a cool place.

In about four weeks the sauerkraut is ready to eat. Each time the container is opened to take out the kraut, the lid, the towel and the stone must be cleaned in boiling water. The inner rim and wall of the container must be kept very clean in order to preserve the fresh flavor of the cabbage.

2. Twenty-five pounds of cabbage, one-third of a cup of sea salt, one-half cup of juniper berries, one-half cup caraway seeds.

Shredded cabbage is pressed into wood or earthenware container, sprinkle corresponding amount of salt, juniper berries and caraway seeds as well as some sliced apples and dill. Repeat layers until container is full with all layers pressed firmly down until juice covers all layers. Proceed with lid, stone and cover as explained above.

After 30 days the finished product will be found to be most tasty and nutritious. Kept in the original container in a cool place, the sauerkraut will keep for several months. Once removed from the container, it should be kept in the refrigerator. As an enticing part of any salad, the fermented cabbage could help to make many a meal more delectable.

The juice is extremely nutritious and of exquisite taste, and slightly laxative.

PICKLED CUCUMBERS (Using Sea Salt)

The salt content is still much less than usually contained in commercial products. The amount is 23 grams per one quart and should be accurately determined by having respective amounts weighed out (46 grams for half gallon, 92 grams for one gallon, etc.) to suit amount planned to be prepared.

The container is a wooden barrel or earthenware crock. Clean with boiling water before use.

Herbs such as dill, laurel, bay, etc., and pieces of horseradish with a few onions and a little garlic will render savory taste.

Small, sturdy cucumbers are soaked 24 hours in cool water, are dried with cloth. Pickles are tightly placed side by side and row upon row into container with no empty spaces permitting. The above mentioned herbs and spices are placed between layers.

The salt solution is brought to a boil, allowed to cool somewhat and poured still hot over cucumbers until fully covered. Cover with clean cloth and over that wooden lid with ventilation holes, on top of which is placed a heavy rock. The container is placed in somewhat warm spot in basement or other location.

The salt solution must extend above the wooden lid. In about thirty days the fermenting process is completed and container can be placed in cool spot. Pickles are now ready to be eaten.

Every fourteen days the cloth, lid and rock must be cleansed, any scum has to be removed.

12

The New Diet
for Dynamic Health

The human race is conditioned by heredity, environment and habits. As such it is obvious, that any change of the deeply ingrained living pattern is subjected to all sorts of reservations, if not downright rejection.

This "restrained enthusiasm" is particularly understandable when the proposed change is direcetd toward Man's primary urge, that of self-preservation. The eating of the customary fare has established powerful conditioned reflexes which may require heroic efforts to be overcome. Fear, doubt and disbelief are the predominant reasons explaining the fact that the new eating approach is not followed by the majority of people.

To do without meat, fish and eggs is preposterous to the mind of many. A pseudo-scientific reasoning is resorted to that meat furnishes "best" protein and that it is "complete" in all of its amino-acids. More potent arguments may be projected such as that it is "essential" to the maintenance of life.

Very few of us know that the green leaves of plants plus the "lowly" potato contain the highest quality protein. These live substances are complete in all amino-acids, in contrast to protein of meat, which lacks three of the amino-acids, besides possessing undesirable side effects formerly discussed.

We should also be reminded that there are *more* people on this globe living *without* than with flesh foods.

It could be argued that many of the vegetarian races do not necessarily demonstrate high degrees of vitality. This is true. The underlying reason for this state of sub-health is *not* the vegetarian eating concept but the subsistance on foods insufficient in amounts, quality or naturalness. In short, some of the less vital races try to get along on a starvation diet.

THE EGG PROBLEM

Admittedly, there are many pros and cons in evaluating this "explosive" subject. The adjective is meant here in a literal sense, as the egg is the beginning of a new life. Its protein content is of extreme, complex nature and subjective to putre-factive changes more violent than observed in flesh eating. As noted in another chapter, the decay bacteria content is many times that of meats.

I have often wondered just why the waste products derived from egg digestion are so hostile to the human organism. We know of the complexities of the purine bodies or uric acids released by all protein digestion which could inaugurate auto-intoxication. But the egg protein is still more deeply involved, as yet not completely understood.

Alkaloids coming from a dead but fully completed or de-veloping animal are known to exert certain damaging effects upon human tissues. But in the egg a different situation is en-countered. Life is presented in latent form—contingent on undergoing rigid provisions for development. *Specific substances* are required to carry on this "ripening" process and it is possible that here we will find the true cause of unpredict-able behavior in the assimilation of eggs.

Further research is needed but for the time being it is ad-visable to be very careful with egg consumption. Two or three eggs per week may be sufficient to be used in connection with preparing other foods such as "breading" for meats, fish, etc.

In my own case, there was a time when I was partial to generous egg intake to "compensate" for the absence of flesh foods. In due time I noticed the development of little horny moles on both of my ankles. The suspicion was directed to-wards the diet and I decided to completely stop the eating of eggs in any form. All skin blemishes disappeared like magic within a period of sixty days.

This cautious "egg-less" orientation was projected into the diet habits of my students. With clockwise precision, similar improvements in skin conditions were noted. In one case, a persistent "wart trouble" seemed to have lessened.

RAW FOOD BENEFITS

Here we find the other pole of resistance to the eating reform. The cooking idea has taken such deep roots that conversions to the fireless method are difficult to achieve.

At the start, a compromise could be made to establish the daily fare on a 50-50 basis. The cooking processs of one-half of the food is altered to a brief steaming of a few minutes, permitting the "survival" of some of the live forces in the plant product. The other half is enjoyed in their natural state.

We should always try to obtain some *green leaves* every day. Live substances are impregnated in this green earth's cover, embodying the secrets of life. There is no other substance available anywhere that can surpass their nutritional value. The chlorophyll which renders the green to the leaves, helps to build strong tissues and blood, and normalizes glandular functions. The green leaf maintains the acid-alkaline balance and with its top grade protein, even in small quantities, supplements the protein of grains. Truly, the green leaf is the connecting link between man and the cosmic forces through the rays of the sun.

WHOLE GRAINS

We have learned that the European nutritional revolution had been sparked by two powerful, but scholarly personalities. One was a physician, Dr. Bircher-Benner of Switzerland, the other a philosophy student searching for health, Are Waerland of Sweden. Both men were adamant in their conviction of plant foods constituting superior nutrition. Grains are the seeds of plants (grasses).

Bircher-Benner reawakened interest in an old grain usage where whole oats furnishes the basis of a delicious breakfast dish, known as the Muesli. Waerland popularized the combination of several whole grains which he termed Kruska.

The Muesli and Kruska are known today to millions in Europe. In both cases the dishes are supplemented with fruit or berries and small amounts of dairy products.

Recently, a German illustrated weekly published an interview with the famous cancer researcher Professor Otto Warburg, recipient of the Nobel prize for medicine. A photograph accompanying the article showed attached to the table in the institute, a small hand mill for grinding whole grains, for the domestic needs of Warburg's co-workers.

Another Nobel prize winner, Dr. Kollath, also "steps back into the past" by shunning the finished product sold in stores and prepares the whole kernels for the family's need.

While it is true that grains do lack two or three amino acids, this loss can easily be corrected by fruits or vegetables, particularly green leaves. One type of food supplements the other, leading up to an entirely different concept of taste satisfaction.

A new realization permeates the individual. To be concerned about one's body and food is of little purpose unless it results in the evolvement and awakening of inner dormant powers. The secrets and potentials of the soul are withheld from those who constantly transgress the laws of sound nutrition.

SALTS AND SPICES

The use of table salt may be greatly reduced, if not entirely discarded.

Sea salt (evaporation process) replaces the former. This applies to the slightly steamed variety of vegetables.

Raw food is prepared *without* any salt. Natural herbs can be used as spices.

DAIRY PRODUCTS

Small amounts of yogurt, buttermilk, sour milk, cottage cheese and other mild cheeses can be well tolerated by the human organism. Lactic acid is the end-product of these fermented dairy products and highly desired in the colon for growth of the right kind of bacteria for the human body.

It must be remembered, however, that dairy products essentially are destined by nature to provide nutrients from a mother animal to its offspring. The specific animal characteristic is imbedded in this product, geared to the respective demand of the growing animal. There exist certain discrepancies as pertaining to mineral and protein content in comparison to human milk. Furthermore there are other important features such as growth hormones, which compel us to use all dairy products in moderation.

SOIL CONDITIONS

The quality of a soil is mirrored in the state of health of its inhabitants. We have learned about the superior soil condition in Deafsmith County.

But there are also many poor soils. Dr. Albrecht demonstrated it pointedly by showing two carrots from different farms. Both carrots looked alike, one was normal in mineral content, but the other was practically devoid of any nutritional value. Albrecht remarked of this: "The decline in soil fertility responds in lowering of health condition of plants, animals and human beings."

Synthetic fertilization is not the answer, the earthworm holds the secret to soil health. In association with bacteria, fungi, etc., a handful of fertile soil virtually quivers, full of life.

Chemicals and synthetics kill this throbbing life force which may have been the reason for the existence of the strange, "lifepoor" carrot. Try to secure fruits and vegetables grown in naturally fertilized soils.

PREPARATION FOR VEGETABLE CLEANSING

For the cleansing of root vegetables no special direction is necessary. The cleansing of leaf vegetables may require a basin with cool water in which a handful of table salt has been dissolved. After an hour or so of soaking, the vegetables are taken out and washed in running water. To counteract worms, or poisonous sprays, the leaves may be spread out in the sun, each side exposed to its rays for a few minutes.

CHOPPING

The chopping up of hard foods of this kind serves two purposes.

1. The production of tasty dishes for the table pleasing to the eye.
2. The accommodation of raw vegetables to human chewing capacities.

Our tooth structures are not what they are supposed to be and outside help is needed.

The more defective the chewing capacity, the more necessary becomes the artificial chopping up of the food.

In our home, we use a Swiss made chopper with multiple knives which works excellently and can be purchased in most health stores.

Even when chopped up by mechanical means, raw food still demands thorough mastication. The blood and the foundation of the teeth are better nourished by raw food, the teeth become hard again and the chewing capacity is increased.

BINDING SUBSTANCES

Some binding substances can be added to improve the nutritional value and the flavor of raw vegetable dishes. They can consist of vegetable oils coming from saf-flower, sesame, sunflower, olive, etc. and freshly squeezed lemon juice. The addition of aromatic herbs is a matter of taste. Fine chopped onions and parsley will always enhance the state and food value of the dish.

In the diet of the Bulgarians, raw onions play a considerable part and the relative rarity of cancer among the population of Bulgaria has been attributed to their plentiful use of onions as food.

THE NEW STEAMING PROCESS

Water should never be permitted to come in contact with the food in the steaming process. Little wire screens are usually

available in health stores which separate the small amount
of water at the bottom of the container from the food. Only a
few minutes are required to slightly change the composition
of the food from the raw to a "mature" state. The destruction
begins even at a temperature of 140°F. and is the more serious
the longer the steaming lasts.

The effect of steaming upon whole potatoes is less harmful.
Young, still unripe potatoes and old seed potatoes should not
be eaten raw as then their relatively high solanine content
might be injurious. Besides steaming, potatoes could be baked
whole or halved, rubbing the skins with butter before placing
in oven.

Besides potatoes there are a number of root vegetables such
as celery, sweet potatoes, etc. that can endure the steaming
process without too much damage.

For a most satisfying meal it is advisable to get a number
of the following vegetables, which can be consumed in their
raw state:

Lettuce, tomato, celery, green peppers, cabbage, cucumber, kohlrabi, carrot, onion, garlic, parsley, watercress, cauliflower, green peas, dandelion greens, avocado, radish, spinach,
beets, endive and zuccini squash. Broccoli, mushrooms and
artichokes should be steamed.

In the form of a salad the vegetables are slightly broken up
in preference to being cut with a knife.

In addition to the salad dressings discussed, the vegetables
can be made more appetizing and still more nutritious by
sprinkling with sesame, sunflower, flax or chia seeds.

ALKALINE FOODS

The "fruitarian" diet is the most sensible way of eating.
Fresh fruits should always command the number one position
in our daily fare. Let us establish the habit of keeping a generous variety of both local and tropical fruits available.

Dried fruits are particularly recommended. Figs, dates,
prunes, etc., should be in every household.

Dried prunes are the most alkaline reacting food known, together with lima beans, olives and spinach. One never tires

of eating prunes. They are indispensable to athletes but still more needed by the plain citizen of sedentary occupation as a natural laxative.

The apple, the king of fruits should be eaten every day in its natural state. Grapes, the queen of fruits are to be enjoyed during their ripening season.

In general, all fruits and vegetables leave an alkaline reaction provided they are eaten in their raw state. This is one of the most pertinent reasons why the raw food diet has been so successful in overcoming difficult interferences to body metabolism.

HOW MUCH FOOD?

The more harmoniously the meals are put together and the more raw food is included—the more economic and effective will it respond in the organism. This internal economy is one of the objectives with this new diet.

Too much food increases neither health nor performance but leads to premature aging and disease. Many European diet experts agree that the average person eats about one-half more than needed.

It is said that a drunkard may die of old age, but a glutton never! Remember that raw food may have forty times the nutritional force of its cooked counterpart. Chew it well, digestion starts at the mouth where the food must be thoroughly mixed with saliva (ptyalin).

CHIA

The latest food sensation coming from the Western parts of North and South America is *chia,* a seed originating from the *genus salvia.* Chia is a seed of a desert plant thriving in sandy soils where abundance of sunshine is prevalent throughout the year. This makes *chia* a typical desert food appreciated by miners, prospectors, Indians, and all of those acquainted with the problem of survival in periods of scarcity. It is said that a teaspoon of *chia* could make a meal of a most delicious nutty flavor. The seeds are very small and are of various shades of gray resembling ground pepper about the size of the alfalfa seed. They are crisp and crunchy when chewed and quickly transform into a mucilaginous consistency. The mineral make-up of the seed as yet has not been scientifically determined but one-fifth of it consists of a first-class protein. The fat content equals that of linseed which in itself explains the extraordinary nutritional value of this delightful food.

There are all sorts of fantastic stories connected with *chia*. In all tales, emphasis is pointed toward longevity and well-being of those partaking of the tiny nutty kernels.

A number of my students also wholeheartedly vouch for the superiority of the little seeds. I am sure you equally will find this natural product most enticing. The re-discovery of this exciting food will benefit all of us.

SEED (NUT) DIGESTION

Seeds contain all ingredients needed for the build-up of a new plant. The main components are proteins, auxones, enzymes and mineral trace elements essential for life creation.

The food substances in seeds are extremely concentrated. A little will go far. If consumed in excess, it will equally respond by undergoing putrefaction Also, if not completely chewed, the gritty nut portions may become retained in the folds of colon pockets, giving rise to decay. Auto-intoxication will then show its mark often displayed by dull aches in back of head.

From this we should learn that the amount of ingested food is important as well as the practice of chewing. In view of our bad teeth, it is almost impossible to chew seeds or nuts as efficiently as they should be. A small mill should be acquired, to grind the nuts to a smooth consistency.

ARE VITAMINS NECESSARY?

This is an often asked question. My answer: "If one knew the sources of food—the type of soil, factors of harvest, etc., and found them satisfactory, if at the same time foods were consumed mostly in their raw state—no food supplement would be required.

Since practically all of these provisions are not in force, vitamin and mineral substances have often helped to overcome serious food deficiencies.

NATURAL VITAMINS

Always insist on obtaining natural concentrates from health stores. The chemical laboratory can never equal or replace the natural vitamin complexities created by plants.

Natural vitamins, under polarized light, show *optical rotation* in contrast to synthetic vitamins which are *optically inactive*. It is the old story about the chemist who can imitate an egg but cannot make it hatch.

Actually, there is no such thing as a synthetic vitamin. Like all foods, it has to come from the soil or the sea, where the life giving properties had been generated from the cosmos, through the rays of the sun.

13

Kruska and Honey for New Energy

Here is a recipe for Kruska, a veritable staff of life:
Equal parts of whole kernels of:

      Rye
      Barley
      Wheat
      Oats

Grind through small mill or blendor; of this take two heaping tablespoons, add raisins and wheat bran according to taste and soak in warm water, a little more than needed to cover amount. Let stand overnight and the following morning put container in double boiler and heat to a little *below boiling.* Place container into "straw box" that is a carton filled with straw or old newspapers, covered with old blanket or pillow. Let stand for at least one hour but preferably three to four hours. The thermos bottle also efficiently serves the purpose, pre-heat bottle first with boiling water before puting in the kruska. The gruel of kruska must still be steaming when taken out of container. It is eaten with a little milk and honey.

This is the fundamental version of Waerland's Kruska, which could be enjoyed at breakfast or lunch. In combination with fruits and alternated with diets of green leaves, stalks and root vegetables, there is *no finer tasting nor more nutritious food found anywhere regardless of the amount of money spent.*

Galenos, famous ancient physician, said that those who wish to remain healthy must not avoid the foods of the common people. How true this is. I have learned that the more expensive the food the more derogatory it is to health.

I am reminded about the old John D. Rockefeller, who lived up to his nineties on a true austerity diet. I do recall a dish of gruel he had taken everyday, which possibly could have been the "live" variety made from whole kernels. I am sure that Mr. Rockefeller could have afforded better foods, if money could have bought it. It is not often that one encounters such a rare combination of wealth and wisdom.

In grasses, we find the highest concentration of food substances per given amount. Have you ever wondered about horses or cattle becoming sleek and sturdy on nothing but the green grass?

Grains are the seeds of grasses and as such the still more concentrated sum total of an already concentrated food.

The proverbial well-being of the people in Scotland could be explained by the "brose," a dish made by pouring boiling water on grains, usually oatmeal.

In Ireland, the dish is called "scalded oats." The rugged vitality of the Russians becomes apparent to anyone visiting their country. The "kaszewarka" is the meal from whole millet, crushed, with boiling water poured over it.

In the Orient we find whole rice giving stamina to people. I have observed dock workers in Japan carrying 200 pound sacks, ten hours a day on a handful of rice with a few leaves of sea kelp.

From all this it can be surmised that grains have been endowed by nature as cornerstones in the building of food provision. Yet there are some in the diet field who reject grains on the ground that "seeds are meant for the birds."

Be it as it may, birds or no birds, it would be impossible to conceive this world without grains to sustain its population in the past or now. That grain products have contributed greatly to the deplorable health deterioration of civilized races is true. It is also understandable that an evolved orientation of "starch awareness" could develop among those of us who were searching for the cause of our physical disorders. The breakdown of the human organism was rightly connected to the consumption of carbohydrates. The term "starch" became the scapegoat for all of the ills suffered.

A great mistake had been made. The baby had been discarded with the bath water.

It is not the grain that is at fault, *but what is done with it.* The big question mark again looms up in front of us. How is it possible that an insignificant minority of people, a mere handful of them, have been and still are permitted "to do that" to man's rightful heritage of obtaining life supporting sustenance? It is the refining process which does all of the damage. It is common knowledge that natural foods contain life forces which will sustain life. It is equally known that the refining process of foods kill these life properties, rendering it sterile, *unable to sustain life.*

Test animals given nothing but refined grains will die sooner than those animals receiving nothing but water.

The profit motive compels the changing of nutritious substances into commodities that could be stored for months or years just as so much *sand or gravel.*

Dead substances no longer can attract bugs or weevils. In a few refined products, where a fraction of live substances have been retained, poisonous chemicals are added for more "preservation."

The grain kernel is protected by a tough outer membrane or shell, which nature intended to constitute effective keeping qualities for years or even centuries. Violate this outer covering, and the contained food substance immediately begins to deteriorate.

So-called enriched bakery products made from refined grain are heaping insult to injury. Again, the proof of the pudding is in the eating. Test animals died sooner on an exclusive diet of "enriched" refined food than other animals fed exclusively on the refined substance. Similar sad results had been observed on tests of refined grain products where "a little life" had been retained. Bugs and weevils soon started to attack this commodity, necessitating the use of more chemicals with increasing toxicity.

All of this, because of an unimpressive tiny, innocent little shell ruthlessly removed. Our lesson? Insist on obtaining *whole kernels of grain,* keep intact until using and "grind" only *enough* as can be consumed each day. The contact of the ground mass with the air brings on the oxidation of vital substances. In about ten days, little, if any live substance is left.

The question may be asked, how is it that people *do* survive in view of all statements made above. The previously discussed order of "half health" is the answer, where people do not "live" but "exist." The twenty to one reserve potential of the human organism permits the body to "creep" along without vitality to an early grave. Furthermore, the octopus of commercial food processing as yet allows a few other foods to dribble through its squeezing tentacles.

VARIATIONS IN PREPARING KRUSKA

There are many interesting variations in which the Kruska or facsimile may be prepared.

Some of my students like the dish better by foregoing the soaking but boiling it for five minutes immediately after the grain has been ground in the small mill. The straw box is then made use of by preventing the container from cooling off too rapidly for a period of from one to three hours.

In another version of this most nourishing grain preparation, the types of grains are interchanged, such as millet, brown rice, wild rice, buckwheat, corn (sweet) or even lentils, split peas, etc., to satisfy specific tastes.

Here is an opportunity for interesting experiments that can be conducted, generally bringing good results.

In this connection it must be pointed out that some of the grains may be harder than others. Oats, barley and buckwheat for instance are decidedly more tender than rye or wheat. Also condition and length of storage of the grains must be considered. In some cases a previous soaking period would definitely help to restore moisture content approximating that of the ripening of the grain.

It is axiomatic that concrete rules can not be established as to right time or soaking requirements of the grain. With a little practice, this most interesting food procurement will quickly establish the correct procedure.

AN EXTRA-VITALITY BREAKFAST

Make a mixture of all available grains such as wheat, barley, rye, oats, buckwheat, millet, add flaxseed, chia, sesame and sunflower seeds and run mixture through mill or blender. A three or four day supply can be made at one time, kept in closed container in refrigerator.

From this take required amount and add dried fruits cut into small pieces. Prunes, raisins, peaches, apricots, dates, figs are used according to taste. In cases of colon sluggishness increase amount of prunes and figs. To this add wheat bran, some wheat germ, comfrey and small amount of brewer's yeast.

Do not cook or heat, only soak in warm water overnight, just enough water to cover total amount.

Some of my students prefer to enjoy the grains and seeds in their whole, unbroken state. In this case they are soaked for 24 hours.

HONEY—THE MIRACLE FOOD

Millions of years before man there were bees on this earth. Possibly the most highly organized type of insect, bees make honey from the pollen of flowers. Pollen is bio-chemically similar to the sexual cells and associated secretions of sex glands of animals. For this reason honey is the only known food which is actually a concentrate of reproductive (sexual) substances. *Honey is rich in enzymes,* so essential for normal digestion and assimilation. Here we find diastase, invertase, catalase, peroxidase, lipase, which provide more natural complexes than can be obtained from "enzymes supplements" with their fancy price tags. *Honey is rich in ionized minerals.* Not only do we find the usual food minerals such as calcium, potassium, magnesium, iron, phosphorus, sulphur, iodine but also the highly impotant trace minerals including boron, chromium, copper, lithium, nickel, titanium and many more.

It must be remembered that the natural bio-chemical (ionized) form in which honey minerals are concentrated are better assimilated than in any other way.

HONEY IS RICH IN ANTI-BIOTICS

It is generally known since ancient times that honey possesses incredible anti-spoiling properties. Even meat used to be preserved in honey. Now research in Russia has revealed high anti-bacteria and anti-mold action in honey. This is why long before penicillin, doctors used honey to heal seriously infected wounds. The anti-biotic factor in honey is immediately destroyed by heat or pasteurization. Heat is equally destructive for the enzymes and ionized state of minerals contained in the honey. Always try to obtain the unheated variety.

HONEY FOR A DYNAMIC LONG LIFE

The sweetening material contained in honey is glucose and levulose. These simple sugars do not require to be digested but are immediately absorbed by the bloodstream as "energy fuel." Indeed, honey could be construed as providing a way to youthful and long life.

The first great doctor, Hippocrates, lived to a ripe old age and ate honey all his life. The famous medical scientist Avicenna said, "If you want to remain young, eat honey."

There are 25,000 men and women in Russia that reportedly have passed the 100-year mark. They have singled out honey for food and medicine more than any other substance—for long life. Honey is used in modern Russian clinics to treat patients with hard to heal sores, nose—mouth—throat ailments, eye diseases, heart diseases, liver and kidney disease, stomach and intestinal ulcers and certain nervous involvements.

The usual daily "dose" is three ounces, in three equal amounts; two hours *before* or three hours *after* meals.

For external conditions, the honey is applied as a poultice.

Recipes
and
Menus

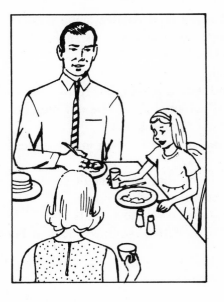

The following recipes are all tested for both palatability and the health factors. One should enjoy one's food while eating.

BASIC NUTRITIONAL RULES

Natural, unchanged food is always the least expensive.
Obtain live food and use it also as such.
Never eat, unless being hungry.
Chew thoroughly.
Eat simple and within reason, but fullworthy and varied.
Our functional potential should be our measure.
Never encourage anyone to eat.
Avoid becoming angry and never create anger in others while eating.
There are no foods that are difficult to digest, but there are wrong combinations and an excess.
Three meals—three bowel movements.
Efficient food assimilation requires sufficient body movements.

14

New Menus
For Healthful Living

THE SPROUTING PROCESS

The maintenance of a medium in the colon consisting of lactic acid has resulted in the recovery of many serious internal degenerations.

Sprouted grains appear to serve this purpose most efficiently. Besides obtaining one-hundred percent raw food, we receive the benefits of pre-digestion. The kernels are easy to chew and very tasty.

Use a wide-mouth mason jar and put in one handful of grains, either mixed or the one of your choice. Soak for twenty-four hours, pour off water and keep moist for three to four days in warm place. Twice daily the grains are inspected, slightly shaken. Little white spots will appear on one corner of the kernels, at which time the sprouts are ready to be consumed. The sprouted grains may be kept in the refrigerator to keep from spoiling. However, it is best to prepare just enough of the seeds to last for one or two days, in which case several jars could be employed to maintain constancy of supply.

Other seeds can also be sprouted in this manner. Foremost of these are seed from alfalfa, soybeans (mung beans), etc.

The above sprouted grains can be mixed with various green leaves and may be consumed whole or after ground in mixer or mill.

RYE GRAINS WITH LEAVES

One cup grains, one-quarter cup nuts, caraway powder, one small onion, some dried herbs or marjoram, thyme or basil.

Rye grains are soaked in water for twenty-four hours then dried (blot with paper towel or in air). Mix all ingredients after grinding grains through mill and cutting up onion.

WHEAT WITH COTTAGE CHEESE

One cup wheat, one cup cottage cheese, green onions or leeks, dill, parsley, two tablespoons oil, salt.

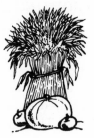

Soak wheat in little water for forty-eight hours, dry and run through mill. Mix with oil and a pinch of salt. Place into deep platter and apply above it to the cottage cheese, which is sprinkled with the finely chopped herbs. Will go well with a raw salad.

SPROUTED WHEAT

Sprout wheat as explained above, and mix with honey or marmalade. Consume whole or run through mill.

WHEAT

One cup of wheat, one-half cup of nuts, one half cup of figs or raisins. Soak wheat 48 hours in water, dry and mix nuts and fruit and run through mill.

BIRCHER MUESLI

Ground oats, one-half lemon, two apples, some nuts and milk.

Oats are soaked 12 hours in enough water to have all of it absorbed. Mix with little milk, juice and peeling of lemon. Apples are grated and immediately mixed into the semi-thick gruel. All is sprinkled with the ground up nuts and consumed. Instead of oats, any or all other grains can be used. Apples may be replaced by other fruits or berries.

CAROB BREAD

Take desired variety of grain, soak for 48 hours, dry by placing between towel, napkins or outside by air and sun for a few minutes.

Use one part kernels, two parts pitted dates, one part raisins, one part figs and put through flaker. Into mixture work as much ground carob meal as it will hold to be rolled to half inch thickness. Cut into convenient small sizes and expose to air and sunshine several hours.

NUT BREAD

Use one part grains soaked 48 hours, dry, add one part almonds, one part brazil nuts, one part hazelnuts. Grind

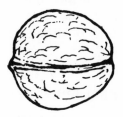

through mill. Mix and sprinkle with a pinch of cinnamon. Spread into thin layers and expose to sunshine for two hours.

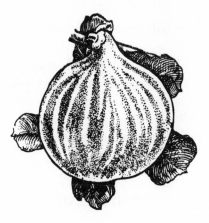

NUT FRUIT BREAD

One part grains of choice or combined, are soaked for 48 hours. Dry and add one part of raisins, one part of dried prunes (stones removed), one part of figs, one part of dates, one part of flaxseed and three parts of nuts of choice. Put through mill, mix and roll into thin layers. Sprinkle sesame seeds on board which will adhere to layers. Cut into small portions. Expose to sunlight for 4 hours.

RAW WHOLE GRAIN BREAD

Use two cups of six varieties of grains, soak 48 hours, dry, put through mill, add one-quarter cup of vegetable oil and enough grape juice to roll into thin layers. Sprinkle sesame seeds on board to prevent sticking as well as making the bread more nutritious. Cut into small sections. Expose to sunshine until dry.

FLAXSEED BREAD (Laxative)

Two cups grains of your choice, all or singular, soak for 24 hours, dry and add one cup powdered flaxseeds, one-half cup nuts, one-half cup raisins, one-half cup sesame or other vegetable oil, one-half cup honey, pinch of sea salt. Run through mill and mix. Roll into layers of half-inch thickness. Slice into narrow sections and put into sunshine to dry.

Note: Whenever sun is not available, the drying process can be attained in oven with *low* heat, keeping door open.

GRAPE DELIGHT

One cup of combination of wheat, oats and barley run through a mill. Soak 12 hours in two cups of grape juice. Mix and knead into bottom of platter. Place on top two cups of grapes with contrasting color such as white and red, garnish with stripes of nut cream.

NUT CREAM

For the sake of convenience, the recipe for this delectable topping is given here.

Any available nuts or seeds may be used. Walnut, brazil, hazel, pine, almond, pecan, sunflower, sesame, watermelon, casaba, etc. The seeds (remember, all nuts are seeds) are placed into a blendor and "triturated" with enough water to make a creamy consistency. The addition of coconuts greatly contributes to improved taste and economy. Coconuts require separate "grinding" in the blendor, as certain woody portions of the liquidized mass must be removed by straining through cloth or strainer. The finished products, together with some natural vanilla extract, plus a little honey, is mixed together. The cream should be prepared immediately before being consumed. Remaining portions may be kept in refrigerator but will separate in a short time and the blendor will have to be employed again before use.

SAUERKRAUT DELIGHT

One cup of mixture of wheat and oats soaked 24 hours in two cups of water with one-half cup of nuts run through a mill.

Add one cup of sauerkraut; one onion, one lemon, a few juniper berries that have been cut up into small pieces. Mix together in a bowl or blendor.

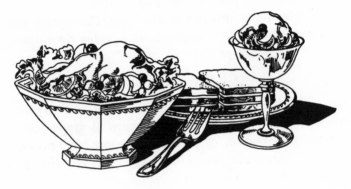

YOGURT VARIATIONS

To the above "delight" can be added yogurt in various amounts, to create more "smoothness."

COTTAGE CHEESE VARIATIONS

Cottage cheese can be added in various amounts according to taste.

Note: Herbal spices such as: sage, cumin, thyme, parsley, marjoram, caraway, bay leaves, onions and garlic do make dishes more delectable. Use according to individual taste.

COTTAGE CHEESE AS SANDWICH FILLINGS

Mix one cup of cottage cheese with one-half cup of yogurt, several chopped green onions, pinch of sea salt and caraway seeds.

COTTAGE CHEESE TRUFFLE

Two cups cottage cheese, one cup nuts, one tablespoon capers, one tablespoon butter, various herbs, and onions, pinch of sea salt, one cup finely chopped celery. All ingredients are well mixed and formed into small balls. Sesame seeds are sprinkled on board on which "balls" are rolled.

COTTAGE CHEESE MAYONNAISE

One cup of cottage cheese is mixed with one-third cup of oil and lemon juice with sufficient amounts of buttermilk or yogurt to achieve creamy consistency. Add onions, sea salt, dill, leeks, some caraway seeds or cumin and marjoram to taste. Mix thoroughly.

There are many delightful combinations in which to mix cottage cheese with herbal spices, yogurt or buttermilk and nut cream. Chopped root vegetables such as parsnips and radishes as well as all other salad vegetables will combine very well. Your own experiments will be rewarding with delectable dishes.

Cottage cheese can also form the main ingredient in sweet or dessert dishes. All kinds of fruit, particularly pineapple and citric variety or grapes, pears or apples can be added, sweetened with honey and spiced with a pinch of cinnamon.

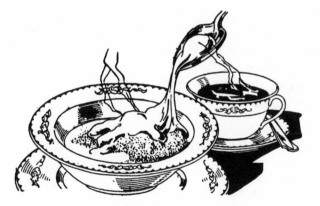

RICE PUDDING

One cup brown or whole rice is soaked 24 hours in water, then drained and thoroughly chopped with one cup of ground almonds or other nuts. Mix into sufficient water to make semi-stiff consistency. Spice with scraped lemon peel, cinnamon and sweeten with honey. The mass is kneaded into flat layers and placed on platters, sprinkled with flaked nuts. Will keep several days in refrigerator.

Whole rice is a tasty and nutritious food. Treated in above manner permits the eating of raw grains in many combinations with cottage cheese, yogurt, honey, various fruits and berries. According to availability of added foods, make your own experiments.

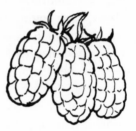

Remember, the soaking of the grain for 24 hours returns enough moisture into the kernels to make them softer, easier to chew and digest. The soaking most nearly re-establishes the consistency of the grain at the time of biological perfection.

The chewing principle should be reviewed in that it *starts* the process of digestion. It is just as important as all implications of *whole food* themselves. Chew until the *mixture is liquid* as only the saliva carries the ptyalin so essential to start complete digestion.

ICE CREAM AND CONFECTION RECIPES

The making of nut cream has been discussed previously. This cream can be made in any desired consistency by the amount of water used in the trituration process of the nuts in the blendor. With this cream as a base, honey or raw sugar could be used as a sweetening agent. Fresh fruit, berries or melon in season may be added. General amount being two-thirds part cream and one-third fruit.

In our home we use a one gallon size electric freezer which requires ice cubes and salt. There is no effort in making such a nutritious and most delectable ice dessert which can easily be stored in the freezing compartment of the average refrigerator or deep freeze unit.

TASTY CONFECTIONS

The ratio is usually one-half nuts and one-half dried fruits. Any kind of nut or seed will do such as walnut, hazelnut, brazil, almond, pecan, pine nut, sesame, sunflower, chia, etc.

The fruit usually consists of figs, pitted dates or prunes, raisins, apricots, peaches, pears, apples, etc. A little extract of pure vanilla will improve the aroma and taste of the confection.

Nuts and fruits are put through a meat grinder and thoroughly mixed. If too dry, a dash of honey may provide sufficient moisture to the combination to allow it being rolled into

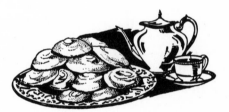

balls. The finished product is then sprinkled with shredded coconut and kept in the refrigerator for future use.

ICE CREAM

The best ice cream is made in the old fashioned freezer, either equipped with electric motor or turned by hand. In most cases, however, this freezing equipment is not usually available and the refrigerator must answer the purpose. Use coldest temperature on dial, place cream in ice tray and beat once or twice during chilling process.

HONEY-NUT ICE CREAM

½ cup honey
½ cup nut pieces
1 cup sweet cream
1 cup nut cream
1 teaspoon pure vanilla extract
Mix dairy cream and nut cream in blendor to add sufficient

air to increase volume (override). Add honey and vanilla and freeze.

AGAR-AGAR HONEY ICE CREAM

Same as above except add agar-agar. This is a pleasant tasting type of seaweed, originally coming from Japan but now being processed from sea vegetation. The addition of agar-agar

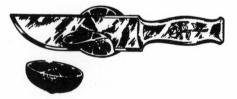

renders not only a gelatinous consistency to desserts or salads, but contributes greatly in nutritional values to the meal.
2 tablespoons agar-agar
1 cup water

The agar-agar flakes are soaked in warm water for five minutes and boiled gently until dissolved (may take 4 minutes). The honey-cream-nut mixture is combined with the agar-agar and beat up in blendor once or twice during the process of freezing.

2 tablespoons agar-agar
½ cup grape juice
½ cup honey
2 cups cut fruit
1 cup sweet cream
1 cup nut cream
½ cup chia seeds
1 teaspoon vanilla
1 teaspoon ground or grated lemon peel
pinch of sea salt

Soak and boil agar-agar until dissolved. Add all ingredients except fruit and triturate in blendor. Add fruit and fill into freezer or ice tray in refrigerator.

BERRY ICE CREAM

½ cup sweet cream
½ cup nut cream
¼ cup honey
1 cup grape or apple juice
Juice of one lemon

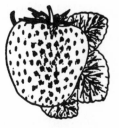

Whip cream in blendor. Blend in other ingredients and add berries. Freeze in ice trays of refrigerator or regular freezer.

COOKED FOOD RECIPES

As formerly indicated, emphasis in this book is placed on naturalness and the raw state of food. However, it is obvious that some foods cannot be completely enjoyed by everyone in their uncooked state. In this category we find potatoes and practically all root vegetables. Also legumes and sometimes grains are difficult to digest without the preliminary cooking process.

Following are a few recipes giving suggestions about delectable dishes that can be prepared with heat. Remember, use as little water as possible. Always try the steaming process first to bring out the delectable flavor of the vegetable.

In the preparation of cereals and legumes water must be used to replenish the moisture of the dried seeds.

Whenever the term salt is used, try to obtain the sea salt variety made from sea water by the vacuum process. Actually the term salt is a misnomer since we are dealing here with ionized minerals which in reality contribute valuable mineral substances to the body economy.

Whenever the terms seasoning, herbs or spices are mentioned, reference is made to aromatic herbs that can be obtained whole or in a powdered state. As suggested in the book, herbs such as sage, marjoram, cumin, garlic, thyme, cinnamon, tumeric, chili, oregano, ginger, paprika, may be used.

Natural, unchanged food is always the least expensive.

CELERY-CARROT-WALNUT LOAF

4 tablespoons butter
¼ cup chopped onion
1 teaspoon sage
½ teaspoon thyme
¼ teaspoon sea salt
2 cups whole-wheat bread crumbs
1½ cups diced celery
1½ cups grated carrots
1 cup nut meats
½ cup cream
2 eggs if desired

Cook onion and other seasonings in butter for two to three minutes. Add bread crumbs, celery, carrots, nut meats and cream. Two eggs well beaten may be added if desired. Mix thoroughly. Bake as a loaf and serve with mushroom sauce.

BEAN CHOWDER

1 cup lima or soy beans
1 medium onion, sliced thin
3 tablespoons butter
seasalt

1 tablespoon minced pimento
Water to cover
1 stalk celery, diced
3 tablespoons diced green pepper

Cook beans slowly until half done. Simmer the onion, pepper, pimento, and celery in the butter for five minutes. Add to beans. Cook slowly until beans are tender. Season.

VEGETABLE-NUT CHOP SUEY

1 stalk celery
1 grated green pepper or pimento
Savita

3 carrots
2 onions
1 cup pecans
1 cup bean sprouts

Steam celery, pepper, and onions for 10 minutes. Add finely chopped carrots and nuts. When almost done add Savita to taste, and then bean sprouts.

MUSHROOM CASSEROLE

2 tablespoons butter
¼ lb. fresh mushrooms or
4 oz. can mushrooms
1 cup brown rice, almost soft
Sea salt to taste.

½ cup grated mild cheese
1 cup cream sauce
1 green pepper chopped
1 med. onion chopped
¼ teaspoon powdered sage

Saute mushrooms and green pepper in butter 5 minutes. Make cream sauce with two tablespoons soy butter, two tablespoons whole wheat flour, 1 cup raw milk. Season to taste. To hot sauce add mushrooms and rice, also onion. Stir and pour into casserole large enough to hold mixture. Top with cheese and sprinkle with paprika. Bake 15 minutes in moderate oven.

CHEESE-NUT LOAF

With 1 pound of cottage cheese mix thoroughly 1 cup of chopped nuts, 1 cup chopped dates and ½ cup chopped ripe olives; season to taste. Place in mold and chill. Serve in slices with raw vegetable or fruit salad. A little honey may be added, if desired, before placing into mold.

NUT MEAT BALLS

¾ cup finely chopped walnuts or other nut meats
½ cup finely ground sunflower seeds
1½ cup cooked millet
2 tablespoons chopped onions
1 tablespoon soy lecithin spread
½ teaspoon mineral or vegetable salt
½ cup finely ground toasted bread crumbs
2 tablespoons finely ground or chopped parsley
⅛ teaspoon curry
⅛ teaspoon cumin
Dash of garlic if desired

Mix all above ingredients. Form into balls. Roll into whole wheat flour. Place in pan and bake 350 degrees F. for about 20 minutes or until brown.

CHICK PEA FOO YUNG

1 cup cooked garbanzos
1 tablespoon chopped onion
6 oz. package of bean or alfalfa sprouts, chopped
1 cup soy cheese
½ cup garbanzo broth
¼ teaspoon mineral or sea salt
1½ tablespoons arrowroot powder

1 tablespoon soy butter
1 teaspoon whole wheat pastry flour
1 teaspoon finely chopped parsley
½ teaspoon ground sage
Dash of garlic

Liquefy soy cheese, arrowroot, soy butter, pastry flour, garbanzo broth and add spices. Add this mixture to the garbanzos, onions, alfalfa sprouts and chopped parsley.

Drop patties on an oiled baking sheet and sprinkle with finely chopped nuts or wheat germ flakes. Bake at 350 degrees F. for about 15 minutes until slightly brown.

EGGPLANT LOAF

Put through grinder one eggplant, one-half cup of nut meats and one onion. Season with sea salt and powdered herbs of choice. Add ½ cup of tomato sauce. Mold into greased loaf pan and bake in a moderate oven for about 15 minutes.

LIMA BEAN LOAF

1 cup cooked lima beans
½ cup green pepper, finely chopped
½ cup whole wheat bread crumbs
½ cup celery, finely chopped
¼ cup onions, finely chopped
½ cup canned mushrooms

1 cup raw cream
½ cup chopped ripe olives
¼ teaspoon powdered sage
4 tablespoons tomato paste
4 tablespoons soy butter (melted)
¼ teaspoon marjoram

Combine all ingredients and put in well oiled loaf pan. Bake in oven for about 20 minutes. Sauce of your choice may be used if desired.

POTATOES WITH CHEESE AND NUTS

3 potatoes diced
½ cup grated cheese
½ cup grated nuts
4 tablespoons soy butter
¼ cup heavy cream

¼ cup chopped parsley
1 cup raw cream
½ teaspoon sea salt
½ teaspoon curry powder
Dash of garlic

Steam the potatoes first and add all other ingredients. Place in baking dish, sprinkle with wheat germ and paprika. Place in moderate oven for about 15 minutes.

CELERY ROOT

2 cups cubed celery root	¾ cup lima beans, cooked
2 tablespoons soy butter, melted	¼ cup chopped parsley
	½ cup grated cheese

Steam celery root until tender. Then combine all ingredients and place in oiled baking dish. Sprinkle with paprika. Bake for about 15 minutes in moderate oven.

COTTAGE CHEESE SALAD

To two cups of cottage cheese add ½ cup grated carrots, ½ cup minced green pepper, ½ cup finely cut red radishes. Add a little onion juice and serve on a bed of watercress, garnished with tomato slices and black olives.

AVOCADO MAYONNAISE

One ripe avocado is triturated in blendor with lemon juice, a little sea salt and powdered herbs of choice.

CABBAGE - CARROT SALAD

1 cup of grated carrots
1 cup of finely chopped cabbage
½ cup of finely chopped celery
1 teaspoon of grated or finely chopped onion

Serve with avocado mayonnaise.

CAULIFLOWER - BEET SALAD

1 cup cauliflower finely chopped
1 cup grated raw beets
1 cup cottage cheese
½ teaspoon finely chopped onion
½ teaspoon finely chopped parsley

Mix and place on lettuce leaves.
May use avocado mayonnaise if you wish.

YAM PUDDING

2 cups cooked yams	1 cup chopped raisins
2 cups chopped apple	½ cup raw cream
1 cup chopped nut meats	1 teaspoon cinnamon

Mix well and pour in buttered shallow loaf pan. Bake uncovered in moderate oven until apples are done and top is brown. May serve hot or cold.

THIRTY DAILY MENUS FOR YOUR HEALTH GUIDANCE

FIRST DAY:
Upon arising a glass of orange juice (⅔ glass of juice, add spring water).

Breakfast:
2 or 3 pears.
Dish of steamed millet with honey and cream.

Luncheon:
Large vegetable salad: Lettuce, cucumber, tomato, avocado, radishes, a few cauliflower blossoms (raw) and black olives.
Season with powdered herbs and sea salt, oil and lemon juice.
If needed—100% whole grain bread and soy spread.

3:00 P.M. Fruit or vegetable drink.

Dinner:
One large baked yam, with soy spread and sea salt.
Small salad: Lettuce, radishes, cucumbers, cottage cheese. Two steamed vegetables—peas and corn, add soy spread and sea salt.
Late evening: Warm carob drink, with whey powder and spring water.

SECOND DAY:
Upon arising—a glass of grape juice (one-third glass, add spring water).

Breakfast:
Dish of sliced bananas with a little cream and honey. Dates stuffed with almond butter.

Luncheon:
Large fruit salad: Pears, apples, grapes and if available a few red cherries to enhance. Serve with or without dressing and whole rye bread with soy spread.

3:00 P.M. Vegetable juice drink or vegetable juice cocktail.

Dinner:
Soup: One cup of green pea soup.
Entree: Cooked lima beans, simmered with onions and sweet green peppers—about 20 minutes.
Small raw salad: Lettuce, cucumber, tomato, avocado.
Two steamed vegetables: one-half green squash and string beans.
Season with soy spread and sea salt.
Late evening: Herbal tea if desired.

214

THIRD DAY:

Upon arising—glass of spring water, add lemon juice—hot or cold.
Breakfast:

A dish of red raspberries (honey if desired).

Toast of whole grain bread and soy spread.

Luncheon:

All the watermelon or other melon you can eat; that is all, nothing can be eaten with melons.

3:00 P.M. Fruit drink.

Dinner:

Large raw salad: Lettuce, parsley, celery, cucumber, tomato, avocado, radishes, olives and cauliflower blossoms (raw) season with favorite dressing and sea salt.

Can have two steamed vegetables such as grated beets and yellow corn with soy spread.

Late evening: Herbal tea with lemon and honey.

FOURTH DAY:

Upon arising, a glass of apple juice (three-quarters juice, add distilled water).

Breakfast:

Large delicious apple—blended in liquifier with cup of raw cranberries and honey to taste.

Whole grain bread with soy spread.

Luncheon:

All the cantaloupe or other melon you can eat—nothing else.

3:00 P.M. Fruit drink.

Dinner:

Large raw salad: Lettuce, celery, cucumber, sweet green pepper, avocado, parsley and alfalfa sprouts. Season with vinegar, salad oil and sea salt.

Small dish of cottage cheese, for extra "zip" add teaspoon of loganberry jam (made with honey).

Late evening: Herbal tea if desired (warm).

FIFTH DAY:

Upon arising a glass of papaya juice (one-half glass juice, one-half glass spring water).

Breakfast:

Large dish of grapes (should have seeds but do not eat the seeds).

Luncheon:

Large apple salad with raisins and pears.

3:00 P.M. Fruit drink.

Dinner:
    Soup: Vegetable soup.
    Large raw salad: Lettuce, sweet green pepper, tomato, cucumber with black olives and favorite dressing.
    Mushroom casserole.
    Steamed peas and carrots.
Late evening: Herbal tea with honey and lemon.

SIXTH DAY:
    Upon arising, a glass of grapefruit juice (two-thirds glass juice, add spring water).
Breakfast:
    Large delicious apple, blended in liquifier with one-half cup carrot. Sprinkle with cinnamon and add honey if desired.
Luncheon:
    Large salad: Grated raw carrot, celery, fresh corn scrapped from cob, lettuce, tomato, avocado. Season with sunflower oil and lemon juice, sea salt to taste.
3:00 P.M. Fruit or vegetable juice.
Dinner:
    Raw salad: Alfalfa sprouts, lettuce, avocado, olives, tomato.
    Nut loaf made from grated carrots, chopped celery, onions, nuts.
    Steamed squash or green chard.

SEVENTH DAY:
    Upon arising, a glass of papaya juice (one-half glass juice, add spring water).
Breakfast:
    Dish of strawberries with honey and cream.
Luncheon:
    One baked potato, seasoned with soy spread and sea salt.
    Raw salad of lettuce, tomato, watercress and radishes.
    Whole grain bread with soy or peanut spread.
3:00 P.M. Vegetable juice.
Dinner:
    Soup: Cup of pea soup.
    Entree: Two slices of vegetable cutlets with onion and sweet green pepper, simmered for 20 minutes.
    Salad of lettuce, cucumber, tomato, celery and black olives.
    Steamed summer squash and green beans.
Late evening: Herbal tea with lemon and honey.

EIGHTH DAY:
    Upon arising, a glass of grape juice (one-half glass juice, add spring water).

Breakfast:
All the delicious apples you can eat with raisins and almonds.
Luncheon:
Large pear salad with cottage cheese.
Whole grain bread with soy or peanut spread and crushed pine-apple, add honey if desired.
3:00 P.M. Fruit juice.
Dinner:
Soy-o-cheese sliced and sauteed in soy spread with onions and sweet green peppers sliced.
Large raw salad: Watercress, cucumber, tomato, radishes, lettuce.
Late evening: Warm juice or herbal tea.

NINTH DAY:
Upon arising, a glass of spring water, add juice of lime.
Breakfast:
Dish of millet (previously soaked) with honey and cream.
Luncheon:
Raw Salad: Lettuce, avocado, tomato, cucumber, watercress.
Baked potato, serve with spread and sea salt.
3:00 P.M.: Vegetable juice.
Dinner:
Salad: Alfalfa sprouts, tomato, lettuce, avocado, spinach (raw).
Lentils steamed until soft with grated onions and finely chopped celery. Add a dash of sage (powdered) for seasoning and sea salt.
Late evening: Carob drink, add honey.

TENTH DAY:
Upon arising, juice of lime with glass of spring water.
Breakfast:
Dish of soaked prunes.
Slice of corn bread with soy spread.
Luncheon:
Small raw salad: Lettuce, grated carrots, raisins, tomatoes, add sunflower oil and lemon juice.
Baked yam with soy spread and sea salt.
Dinner:
Large raw salad: Chopped fresh spinach, alfalfa sprouts, avocado, tomato, lettuce.
Nut loaf with mushroom sauce.
String beans with vinegar and oil dressing.
Late evening: Apple juice, hot or cold.

ELEVENTH DAY:
Upon arising, a glass of orange juice (two-thirds glass juice, add spring water).

Breakfast:
   One or two fresh peaches eaten from hand.
   Dish of steamed whole grain brown rice, honey and cream.
Luncheon:
   All the watermelon you can eat, nothing else.
3:00 P.M.: Fruit or vegetable juice.
Dinner:
   Large raw salad: Alfalfa sprouts, avocado, watercress, tomato, lettuce.
   Baked potato, steamed cauliflower and string beans.
Late evening: Glass of grape juice (one-half glass juice, add water).

TWELFTH DAY:
   Upon arising, a glass of black cherry juice (two-thirds glass juice, add spring water).
Breakfast:
   A dish of fresh cherries or berries.
Luncheon:
   Two or three peaches with dried fruits, two dates, handful of raisins, two figs or dates stuffed with raw ground nuts.
3:00 P.M.: Fruit juice.
Dinner:
   Cream of asparagus soup (made in blender or liquifier).
   Two cutlets (Miller's), simmered with onions and sweet green peppers. Raw vegetable salad: Romaine lettuce, avocado, dandelion greens (raw), olives. Serve with favorite dressing.
Late evening: Fruit drink.

THIRTEENTH DAY:
   Upon arising, glass of apple juice (two-thirds glass juice, add spring water).
Breakfast:
   Kruska with raisins, honey and cream.
Luncheon:
   Salad: Alfalfa sprouts, spinach, avocado, lettuce, radishes.
   Vegetable slightly steamed, corn on cob or string beans.
3:00 P.M.: Vegetable juice cocktail.
Dinner:
   Corn chowder
   Large raw salad
   Baked yam or potato.
Late evening: Peppermint tea, add honey.

FOURTEENTH DAY:
   Upon arising a glass of prune juice (two-thirds glass of juice, add spring water).

Breakfast:

Dish of strawberries with honey, add a little cream.
Two slices of seven grain toast with soy spread.

Luncheon:

Large fruit salad: Pears, apples, grapes and if available a few red cherries to enhance. Serve with or without dressing and whole rye bread with soy spread.

3:00 P.M. Fruit juice.

Dinner:

Soup: One cup of lima beans or green pea soup.
Vegetable salad with favorite dressing.
Nut loaf with mushroom sauce.

Late evening: Herbal tea of your choice.

FIFTEENTH DAY:

Upon arising, a glass of orange juice (two-thirds glass of juice, one-third spring water).

Breakfast:

Two delicious apples with dried fruits such as two figs, two dates, handful of raisins and a few walnuts.

Luncheon:

Salad: One cup alfalfa sprouts, three-quarters cup of lima beans, one-half sliced avocado, tomato—serve with favorite dressing.

3:00 P.M.: Fruit juice of choice.

Dinner:

Soup: Vegetable.
Eggplant and brown rice (cut up eggplant and add to simmered onion).
Salad: Lettuce, radishes, onions, olives, cottage cheese.

Late evening: Carob drink, add honey.

SIXTEENTH DAY:

Upon arising, a glass of orange juice (two-thirds glass juice, add spring water).

Breakfast:

Kruska with honey and cream.

Luncheon:

Large pear salad.
Whole grain bread with soy spread and crushed raspberries (if in season) and honey.

3:00 P.M.: Grape juice (one-third glass water).

Dinner:

Lentil soup.
Salad: Alfalfa sprouts, grated beets, tomato, cucumber, olives.
Steamed broccoli and potato.

Late evening: Peppermint tea, add honey.

SEVENTEENTH DAY:
Upon arising, glass of apple juice (two-thirds glass juice, add spring water).
Breakfast:
Dish of soaked prunes.
Slice of corn bread with soy spread.
Luncheon:
Small raw salad: Lettuce, grated carrots, raisins, nuts.
Sliced ripe papaya (one-half medium papaya).
3:00 P.M.: Fruit juice.
Dinner:
Baked sweet pepper stuffed with brown rice (steamed) and season with simmered onions.
Serve with lettuce, tomato and cottage cheese.
Late Evening: Warm carob with honey.

EIGHTEENTH DAY:
Upon arising, a glass of spring water, add juice of lime.
Breakfast:
Dish of millet (previously soaked) with honey and cream.
Luncheon:
Raw salad: Lettuce, avocado, cucumber, watercress, radishes.
Mushrooms with onions.
3:00 P.M.: Vegetable juice.
Dinner:
Corn chowder—chop up raw potato with sliced onions and celery. Add two tablespoons of soy spread and a little cream. Add sea salt. Cook in top of double boiler. Add two cups of corn cut off cob. Add two tablespoons of soy spread and a little cream. Add sea salt.
Late evening: Vegetable juice cocktail (hot or cold).

NINETEENTH DAY:
Upon arising, a glass of black cherry juice (two-thirds glass juice, add spring water).
Breakfast:
Dish of strawberries with honey and cream.
Luncheon:
A dish of cottage cheese with sliced pears.
A dish of prunes (soaked).
Whole grain bread and soy spread.
3:00 P.M.: Fruit drink.
Dinner:
Soup: Asparagus.
Salad: Large raw.

Two steamed vegetables, potato and beans.
Late evening: Peppermint tea, add honey.

TWENTIETH DAY:

Upon arising, a glass of apple juice (two-thirds glass juice, one-third glass spring water).
Breakfast:
Kruska with raisins, add a little honey and cream.
Luncheon:
All the watermelon you can eat, nothing else.
3:00 P.M.: Fruit juice.
Dinner:
Nut loaf.
Salad: Alfalfa sprouts, avocado, lettuce, tomato.
One steamed vegetable.
Late evening: Herbal tea of choice.

TWENTY-FIRST DAY:

Upon arising, a glass of fresh orange juice (two-thirds glass juice, add spring water).
Breakfast:
Dish of berries with apple sauce.
Liquefy in blender, add honey to taste, also sprinkle with cinnamon.
Whole wheat toast and soy spread, honey if desired.
Luncheon:
All the cantaloupe you can eat—nothing else.
3:00 P.M.: Fruit juice.
Dinner:
Cup of vegetable soup.
Two vegetarian steaklets warmed in their own gravy.
Salad: Small raw salad: Romaine lettuce, watercress, parsley, cucumber, beets (grated), tomato.
Late evening: Mint tea and honey.

TWENTY-SECOND DAY:

Upon arising, a glass of grape juice (one-half glass juice, add spring water).
Breakfast:
Dish of fresh figs.
Luncheon:
Vegetable soup.
Salad: Tossed green with your favorite dressing.
Baked potato with soy spread.
3:00 P.M.: Vegetable juice.

Dinner:
  Large vegetable salad.
  Garbanzo beans, steamed chard.
Late evening: Mint tea with lemon juice and honey.

TWENTY-THIRD DAY:
  Upon arising, a glass of spring water and juice of one-half lime
  or lemon.
Breakfast:
  Raw apple sauce, blended with soaked raisins, add cream if
  desired.
Luncheon:
  One ripe persimmon and two pears.
  One-half cup nuts.
3:00 P.M.: Fruit juice.
Dinner:
  Bean chowder.
  Sweet corn on the cob.
  Large vegetable salad.
Late evening: Prune juice (one-half glass juice, one-half glass
  spring water.)

TWENTY-FOURTH DAY:
  Upon arising, a glass of grapefruit juice (two-thirds glass juice,
  add spring water).
Breakfast:
  Kruska with raisins or dates, with honey and cream.
Luncheon:
  Watermelon, all you can eat.
3:00 P.M.: Vegetable juice.
Dinner:
  Cream of asparagus soup (made in blender or liquifier).
  Vegetable-Nut Chop Suey.
  Salad: Small green tossed salad.
Late evening: Vegetable juice cocktail.

TWENTY-FIFTH DAY:
  Upon arising, a glass of berry juice (two-thirds glass juice, add
  spring water).
Breakfast:
  Several sweet plums and if not enough, eat a banana. Add dates
  stuffed with peanut butter if still hungry.
Luncheon:
  Apple and raisin salad.
  Whole wheat bread and soy spread.
3:00 P.M.: Fresh fruit drink.

Dinner:
  Soup: Vegetable.
  Salad: Lettuce, watercress, avocado, tomato, onion.
  Cheese-Nut Loaf.
Late evening: Glass of celery and carrot juice.

TWENTY-SIXTH DAY:
  Upon arising, a glass of fresh orange juice (two-thirds glass juice, add spring water).
Breakfast:
  One or two free-stone peaches.
  Dish of brown rice, honey and cream.
Luncheon:
  Prune and orange salad.
  Slice of whole wheat toast with soy spread.
3:00 P.M.: Vegetable juice.
Dinner:
  Soup: Split pea.
  Salad: Alfalfa sprouts, avocado, cottage cheese, tomato.
  Lentil loaf: Chopped celery, carrots, onions, parsley. Season with sage (powdered) and sea salt.
Late evening: Herbal tea with lemon and honey.

TWENTY-SEVENTH DAY:
  Upon arising, a glass of fresh orange juice (two-thirds glass juice, add spring water).
Breakfast:
  Dish of millet, honey and cream.
  Millet should be soaked overnight. Steam over double boiler until soft.
Luncheon:
  Large fruit salad: Pears, grapes, apples and bananas. Add a cherry or two for color.
  Toast: Whole grain with soy spread.
3:00 P.M.: Papaya juice.
Dinner:
  Soup: Corn chowder.
  Large raw salad.
  Baked yam or potato.
  Steamed chard.
Late evening: Apple juice, hot or cold.

TWENTY-EIGHTH DAY:
  Upon arising, a cup of alfalfa-mint tea, add honey.
Breakfast:
  Kruka with raisins, add honey and cream.

Luncheon:
>Large salad: Grated raw carrot, celery, fresh corn scraped from cob, lettuce, tomato, avocado. Season with sunflower oil and lemon juice. Add sea salt to taste.

3:00 P.M.: Vegetable juice.

Dinner:
>Chick Pea Foo Yung.
>Salad: Green tossed salad, with your favorite dressing.
>Two steamed vegetables: String beans and chard.

Late evening. Herbal tea, with honey

TWENTY-NINTH DAY:

Upon arising, a glass of orange juice (two-thirds glass juice, add spring water).

Breakfast:
>Dish of soaked prunes.
>Slice of corn bread with soy spread.

Luncheon:
>Baked Yam.
>Salad: Grated steamed beets, lettuce, carrots, cabbage. Season with carrot oil and lemon juice.

3:00 P.M.: Berry juice.

Dinner:
>Mushroom Casserole.
>Small vegetable salad.
>Steamed fresh corn and squash.
>Baked potato, if desired.

Late evening: Fruit or vegetable juice.

THIRTIETH DAY:

Upon arising, a glass of spring water with lemon juice and honey. May be hot or cold.

Breakfast:
>Two persimmons.
>One slice corn bread with soy spread.

Luncheon:
>Potato soup.
>Green salad.
>Slightly steamed asparagus and string beans.

3:00 P.M. Mixed vegetable juices.

Dinner:
>Vegetable soup.
>Salad: Equal parts of carrots (raw or slightly cooked) and green peas through food chopper. Add finely chopped watercress and parsley. You may use yogurt or mayonnaise and sprinkle with paprika. Place on lettuce leaves. Add a few olives.

Late evening: Herbal tea, with honey.

15

How to Select
Healthful Food Combinations

In preparing our meals does it matter in which way they are combined? The old menus of roasts, gravy, potatoes, vegetables, pie, coffee and so on; the breakfast of fried eggs, bacon or ham, toast, jam, coffee—are they combined to give us what we expect from our food?

Without becoming too technical or fanatical, we have to admit that some meals make us feel better than others. Could it be because of bad combination of the foods? Let us see.

Starches and sugars require an alkaline medium for digestion, the process of which actually starts in the mouth where ptyaline, a starch-splitting enzyme, is provided in the saliva. Proteins, on the other hand, require an acid reaction in the digestive fluids for their assimilation.

This means that the meat or cheese sandwich is a poorly combined fare and may for this reason be partly responsible for the condition we are in.

Starch foods and sugars should never be eaten together with such proteins as meat, cheese and nuts. Starches and sugars may be combined with vegetables. Do not mix sweet fruits (figs, dates, bananas) with acid fruits (lemons, oranges, grapefruits, pineapple, etc.) Eat each group separately. Milk combines poorly with anything and should be consumed separately.

It has been my experience that it is difficult to adhere strictly to food regulations. In our own home, we do the best we can and let it go at that. Thorough chewing should always be practiced to make up for the laxity in observing the rules of combining foods.

The odor of stools quite often indicates the extent of adherence to chemically correct combinations of foods. If the odor is extremely offensive, poor combination may be the cause. It may also be the result of insufficient mastication.

PROTEIN

Protein foods are those that contain a high percentage of protein in their make-up. Chief among these are the following:

Nuts (most)
Dry beans
Dry peas
Soy beans
All fresh foods (except fat)
Cheese
Olives
Avocados
Milk (low protein)

CARBOHYDRATES

The carbohydrates are the starches and sugars. They are broken up into three groups in the following classification—starches, sugars and syrups, and sweet fruits.

Starches
All cereals
Dry beans (except soy beans)
Dry peas
Potatoes (all kinds)
Chestnuts
Mildly Starchy
Cauliflower
Beets
Carrots
Rutabaga
Salsify
Syrups and Sugars
Brown sugar
White sugar
Milk sugar
Maple syrup

Peanuts
Hubbard squash
Banana squash
Pumpkin
Caladium root
Jerusalem artichokes
Cane syrup
Honey
Sweet Fruits
Banana
Date
Fig
Raisins
Thompson and Muscat grapes
Prune
Sun-dried pear
Persimmon

FATS

The fats are all fats and oils, as follows:

Saf-flower oil
Olive oil
Soy oil
Sunflower seed oil
Sesame oil
Corn oil
Avocados
Butter
Cream

Nut oils
Butter
Substitutes
  cotton seed oil
Pecans
Most nuts
Fat meats
Lard
Tallow

Acid Fruits

Most of the acids eaten as foods are acid fruits. Chief among these are:

Orange
Grapefruit
Pineapple
Pomegranate

Tomato
Lemon
Lime
Sour apple

Sour grape
Sour peach
Sour plum

Sub-Acid Fruits

The sub-acid fruits are as follows:

Fresh fig
Pear
Sweet cherry
Papaya

Sweet peach
Sweet apple
Apricot
Sweet plum

Huckleberry
Mango
Mangosteen
Cherimoya

Non-Starchy and Green Vegetables

Into this classification fall all succulent vegetables without regard for their color, whether green, red, yellow or white. Chief among these are:

Lettuce
Celery
Endive (French)
Chicory
Cabbage
Cauliflower
Broccoli
Brussels sprouts
Collards
Spinach
Dandelion
Beet tops (green)
Turnip tops
  (green)
Chard

Okra
Cow-slip
Chinese cabbage
Chive
Mustard
Dock (sour)
Turnip
Kale
Mullein
Green corn
Eggplant
Green beans
Cucumber
Kohlrabi
Sorrel

Parsley
Rhubarb
Watercress
Onions
Scallions
Leeks
Garlic
Zuccini
Escarole
Cardoon
Bamboo sprouts
Broccoli-de-Rappe
Summer squash
Radish
Sweet pepper

Melons

The melons are as follows:

Watermelon	Casaba	Crenshaw melon
Muskmelon	Cantaloupe	Christmas melon
Honeydew	Pie melon	Persian melon
Honey balls	Banana melon	Nutmeg melon

FOOD COMBINATIONS

Common Foods	Combine Best with	Combine Badlly with
Sweet—fruits (sub-acid)	Milk (sweet or sour)	Acid fruits, starches Cereals, bread, potatoes Proteins
Acid fruits	Other acid fruits— fair with nuts, fair with milk	Sweet (all kinds) Starches (cereals, bread potatoes, proteins) (except nuts)
Green vegetables	All proteins All starches	Milk Fruits
Starches	Green vegetables Fats and oils	All proteins All fruits Acids, sugars
Meats (all kinds)	Green vegetables	Milk, starches, sweets Other proteins Acid fruit and vegetables Butter, cream, oils, lard
Nuts (most varieties)	Green vegetables acid fruits	Milk, starches, sweets Other proteins, acid foods Butter, cream, oils, lard
Eggs	Green vegetables	Milk, starches, sweets Other proteins, acid foods Butter, cream, oils, lard
Cheese	Green vegetables	Starches, sweets, other proteins, acid foods Butter, cream, oils, lard
Milk	Best taken alone, fair with fruits	All proteins, starches Green vegetables
Fats, oils, butter, cream, lard	All starches, green vegetables	All proteins

FOOD COMBINATIONS (Cont.)

Common Foods	Combine Best with	Combine Badlly with
Cereals (all kinds)	Best eaten alone	All foods
Melons (all kinds)	Green vegetables, butter	Acid fruits, all proteins All sweets, milk
Legumes, beans and peas (except green beans)	Green vegetables	All proteins, all sweets Milk, fruits (all kinds) Butter, cream, oils, lard

Index